Public Mental Health

Perspectives and Prospects

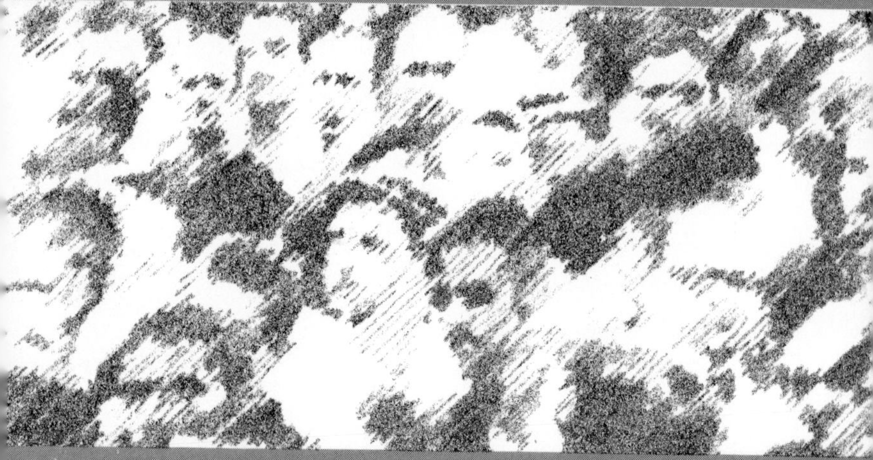

edited by

Morton O. Wagenfeld, Paul V. Lemkau, *and* Blair Justice

Jules V. Coleman, Ernest M. Gruenberg, William G. Hollister, Judith H. Jacobs, Morton Kramer, Alan David Miller, Lucy D. Ozarin, Nolan E. Penn, Darrel A. Regier, Dwight W. Rieman, Norman Sartorius

PUBLIC MENTAL HEALTH

Sage Studies in Community Mental Health 5

SAGE STUDIES IN COMMUNITY MENTAL HEALTH

Series Editor: **Richard H. Price**
Community Psychology Program,
University of Michigan

SAGE STUDIES IN COMMUNITY MENTAL HEALTH is a book series consisting of both single-authored and co-authored monographs and concisely edited collections of original articles which deal with issues and themes of current concern in the community mental health and related fields. Drawing from research in a variety of disciplines, the series seeks to link the work of the scholar and practitioner in this field, as well as advance the state of current knowledge in community mental health.

Volumes in this series:

1. Gary VandenBos (Editor): *PSYCHOTHERAPY: Practice, Research, Policy*
2. Cary Cherniss: *STAFF BURNOUT: Job Stress in the Human Services*
3. Richard F. Ketterer: *CONSULTATION AND EDUCATION IN MENTAL HEALTH: Problems and Prospects*
4. Benjamin H. Gottlieb (Editor): *SOCIAL NETWORKS AND SOCIAL SUPPORT*
5. Morton O. Wagenfeld, Paul V. Lemkau, and Blair Justice (Editors): *PUBLIC MENTAL HEALTH: Perspectives and Prospects*

Additional Volumes in Preparation

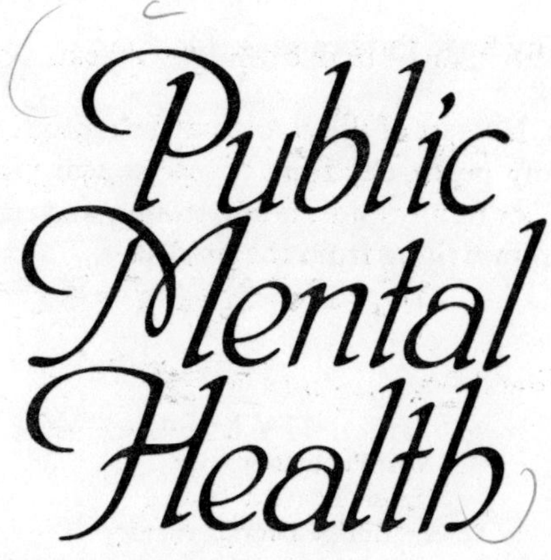

Perspectives and Prospects

edited by

Morton O. Wagenfeld
Paul V. Lemkau
Blair Justice

Volume 5, Sage Studies in Community Mental Health

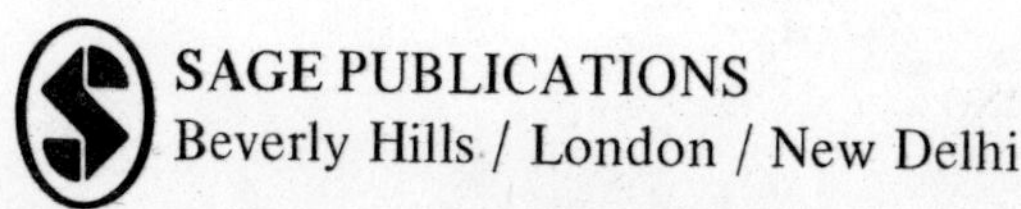

For information address:

SAGE Publications, Inc.
275 South Beverly Drive
Beverly Hills, California 90212

SAGE Publications India Pvt. Ltd.
C-236 Defence Colony
New Delhi 110 024, India

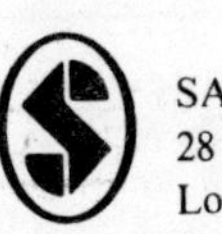

SAGE Publications Ltd
28 Banner Street
London EC1Y 8QE, England

Printed in the United States of America

Library of Congress Cataloging in Publication Data

Main entry under title:

Public mental health.

(Sage studies in community mental health ; v. 5)
Includes bibliographies.
1. Mental health services—United States. 2. Mental health policy—United States. I. Wagenfeld, Morton O. II. Lemkau, Paul Victor, 1909- III. Justice, Blair. IV. Series.
RA790.6.P797 1982 362.2'0973 82-10702
ISBN 0-8039-1120-3
ISBN 0-8039-1224-2 (pbk.)

FIRST PRINTING

Contents

Series Editor's Preface

The community mental health movement has drawn many of its central concepts from the field of public health. In particular, the concern with entire populations, the orientation to prevention, and the communitywide epidemiological perspective are all conceptual frameworks drawn from public health. There is little doubt that community mental health owes a deep intellectual debt to the field of public health. Many of the leaders of the field have now come together to examine the last 25 years in public mental health and to look ahead at the next quarter-century.

The present volume includes a number of papers presented at the observance of the 25th anniversary of the Mental Health Section of the American Public Health Association. Additional chapters have been commissioned especially for this volume as well. These chapters consider the past accomplishments of public mental health and the social and scientific challenges that lie ahead.

Some of the successes of the public mental health movement are documented in this volume. The development of the community mental health center system was due in no small part to the vision of public health-oriented scientists in government agencies such as the National Institute of Mental Health. Today, the more than 700 community mental health centers in existence have permanently altered the pattern of mental health service delivery in the United States. Other efforts of the community mental health movement have not yet been as successful. Attempts to place institutionalized mental patients in communities have met with serious problems of community acceptance and difficulties in providing adequate care. The problem of deinstitutionalization presents a continuing dilemma for public mental health and community mental health in general. At the same time, mental health epidemiology appears to have entered a new era. The Epidemiological Catchment Area studies now underway promise to offer us much more precise information about the prevalence of psychological disorder in the community.

The editors and contributors to this volume survey all of these developments and more. They look to the future and identify a number of emerging issues, including demographic shifts in our population that will produce a new range of health and mental health problems with which we must cope. They also document new efforts to integrate health and mental health services. This organizational and policy development, while looked upon with optimism by some, will require careful scrutiny if the public is to be the ultimate beneficiary.

This is a valuable volume for many audiences. The contributors and editors represent a broad array of disciplines including sociology, psychology, public health, and social work. Scientists interested in future direction for mental health research will find new insights and findings in this volume. Administrators concerned with developing new patterns of care in the field of health and mental health will also find much that is helpful. Finally, those who are teaching the next generation of researchers, treatment personnel, and policymakers in the field of public mental health will find this a useful text for their students. It is, after all, they who will face the scientific and social challenges of public mental health in the years to come.

–Richard H. Price

Acknowledgments

In 1980, the Mental Health Section of the American Public Health Association celebrated its 25th Anniversary. As part of the observance, two scientific sessions were held at the meetings in Detroit to examine some of the major issues in public health of the previous quarter-century, as well as to consider future trends of these issues into the next century. The scholarly and provocative nature of these presentations suggested to a number of us that a more comprehensive treatment of public mental health was in order. Several of the chapters published here are revisions of papers originally presented in Detroit; others were commissioned especially for this volume. Like the field of public mental health itself, contributors to the scientific sessions and to this volume come from a variety of disciplines: public health, psychiatry, psychology, social work, psychiatric nursing, and sociology.

Much of the planning for the Silver Anniversary was done under the aegis of a committee headed by Therese LaLancette. She was assisted by Bertram Black, J. Wilbert Edgerton, Ruth Knee, Judith Jacobs, Paul V. Lemkau, Mabel Ross, and Morton O. Wagenfeld (ex officio). We would like to express our appreciation for the committee's time and effort over the year and, in particular, the dedication, attention, and patient good humor displayed by its Chair. Lois W. Gage and Tom Plaut chaired the scientific sessions and willingly lent their knowledge of public mental health to the task. We are grateful to them for all of their work. William Burian and Laurence T. Cagle read parts of the manuscript and made a number of helpful comments.

The development of this book owes much to the support and encouragement of Richard Price, the Series Editor, and to the good people at Sage. We are grateful to them. Finally, the contributors to this volume are due a particular note of thanks. Their dedication to public mental health may be inferred from their willingness to produce these chapters under sometimes difficult circumstances.

—M.O.W.

Overview

The public mental health perspective is one that is less familiar and, consequently, often less appreciated and understood than its clinical counterpart. It holds a number of principles in common with its parent discipline of public health. The first is a concern with the primacy of preventing disorder and promoting health. The second is a focus on and responsibility for a community or population. This concern with communities requires a multicausal approach, with input from a number of disciplines; public mental health is by nature interdisciplinary. The population or community focus is complementary to the individual orientation characteristic of the clinical perspective. Rather than being antithetical, they complement one another.

This volume examines public mental health in terms of a series of issues and from a variety of perspectives. These several approaches underscore and illuminate the richness and diversity of the field.

The first three chapters deal with the evolution of public mental health within public health from several perspectives. Lemkau traces its origins from the healing temples of ancient Greece, through the Middle Ages, the colonial era, the social reforms of the 19th century, and up to the middle of this century. Ozarin examines the public health/mental health linkage from the federal perspective, seeing its origins in the early concern of the Public Health Service with the problems of mental disorder among immigrants. Her long service with NIMH

Editors' Note: This volume is not an official publication of the American Public Health Association. Identification of the APHA here and in other places in this book is purely for historical purposes. The views expressed by the contributors and editors are their own and do not represent those of the APHA.

affords her a unique perspective on the development of public mental health efforts in the post-World War II period. The most significant development in public mental health, both in terms of expenditures of resources and manpower and alteration of the service delivery system, has been the community mental health centers (CMHC) program. Aspects of community mental health are dealt with by both Lemkau and Ozarin. The chapter by Wagenfeld and Jacobs focuses specifically on CMHCs, considering the sociocultural milieu of the 1960s from which they developed, their legislative evolution, patterns of growth, and probable future.

PROJECTIONS FOR YEAR 2005

Epidemiology is the research and scientific arm of public health. Although not as well known as infectious or chronic disease epidemiology, the epidemiology of mental disorders has made substantial contributions to our knowledge of etiologies. Using J. N. Morris's well-known frame of reference, Regier reviews the major developments in psychiatric epidemiology, particularly over the past 25 years. Kramer's chapter illustrates one aspect of the epidemiological approach. Utilizing morbidity and mortality data in conjunction with population projections, he draws some disturbing conclusions about the nature and prevalence of serious mental disorders into the next century. As mental health professionals, we frequently consider our findings and recommendations to be self-evident and of signal import. That this view is often not shared by others, particularly policymakers, is cause for consternation. Sartorius considers the relationship between epidemiological data and the formulation of mental health policy, particularly the impediments to the utilization of such data.

The community mental health centers program created a need for unprecedented numbers of mental health professionals and paraprofessionals to staff programs. The chapters by Penn and Rieman consider developments of the past 25 and the next 25 years in the training and use of personnel.

As noted earlier, the prevention of disorder is a sine qua non of the public health approach. The prevention of mental disorders was one of the stated goals of the community mental health movement. The vagueness and global nature of many of the early claims made by the proponents of prevention also helped to make it a highly controversial field. The chapters by Lemkau and Justice present rather different and complementary perspectives. Lemkau, adopting a biosocially oriented life cycle approach, argues that the basis for the prevention of mental disorders lies primarily in efforts to avoid the loss of capacities for behavior during the course of development from the fertilized ovum to the end of life. This approach permits interventions targeted to specific disorders or life circumstances. Justice hews to a social-psychologically oriented perspective and also points to the need for very clear specification of the dependent variable—what is to be prevented—and the criteria of scientific rigor necessary for demonstrating the efficacy of prevention efforts. He also cites examples of successful prevention programs.

CHANGES IN SERVICE DELIVERY

In the past quarter-century there have been a number of salient issues in the delivery of public mental health services. Although they did not arise de novo, the rapid expansion of the service system has required more intensive and careful examination of their significance and consequences. Hollister's chapter sets the stage by considering, in a general way, how our strategies of service delivery have changed and "matured" during the period of CMHC expansion and growth. Six areas of change are discussed: service delivery strategy and scope, treatment modalities, consultation strategies, prevention, educational interventions, and administration. It is worth noting that he concludes by observing that we, as public mental health professionals, have also changed and grown in our own outlook and training.

Although mental health has been separated from the general health system for some time—at both the public health and clinical care levels—a persuasive body of epidemiological evidence indicates that most care for mental disorders is rendered in the general medical sector. Recognizing this, the President's Commission on Mental Health (PCMH), in their 1978 Final Report, called for closer ties between the two systems. The ramifications of this linkage is a major concern for public health. Coleman's chapter discusses a number of conceptual models of services linkage and examples of successful programs, as well as some of the problems and difficulties to be encountered in the process of developing liaisons.

One of the spurs to the development of community-based services was the widespread belief that the public mental hospital system had deteriorated to the deplorable state of human warehousing. By 1955, the census in these hospitals had reached its peak and had begun to decline. The community mental health centers movement would accelerate the process of bringing patients out of the hospital and treating them more proximally in the community. This humanitarian concern, buttressed by empirical evidence of the deleterious consequences of long-term hospitalization, helped launch what has become known as the "deinstitutionalization movement." Gruenberg, whose identification of the "Social Breakdown Syndrome" was an important theoretical formulation in the field, critically examines the history and process of deinstitutionalization and some of the myths surrounding it.

The mantle of seer or prophet is one that is exceedingly difficult to don. All of the chapters in the volume deal, in different ways, with one or more aspects of the future of public mental health: the nature of the service delivery system, patient loads, prevention, and manpower and training. Miller's vision of the future is painted with a broader brush on a larger canvas in asking us to consider the problems faced by a meeting of the Mental Health Section of APHA in 2005—the occasion of the 50th anniversary.

Our "Summary and Epilogue" involves a different type of prophecy. In it, we synthesize the major themes articulated in the several chapters, put them in the context of some additional conceptual and economic issues, and use this as background for developing a specific agenda for public mental health.

The Editors

Part I

EVOLUTION AND DEVELOPMENT OF PUBLIC MENTAL HEALTH

Chapter 1

THE HISTORICAL BACKGROUND

PAUL V. LEMKAU

THE MENTALLY ILL AS A PUBLIC RESPONSIBILITY

The care of the mentally ill has, at least since Plato's time, been considered a public duty, to some extent a government responsibility. While maintaining that the care of the mentally ill was the responsibility of the family, the power to enforce such care was placed in the government in Plato's utopian "Republic" (Lewis, 1941). Earlier, Hippocrates had tied mental illness to the field of medicine very securely, as seen in his concept of epilepsy, then considered a mental disease. "It (epilepsy) thus appears to me to be in no way more divine, nor more sacred than other diseases, but has a natural cause from which it originates like other affections" (Zilboorg, 1941). This attitude was strongly resisted by many scholars who tended to separate "naturally caused" diseases of the body from the mind-caused (mind often meant supernatural) mental illnesses. Medical and government (public) responsibility in the field of mental illnesses are thus seen as being mutually involved in the care of the mentally ill since the earliest recorded history.

THE SEPARATION OF THE MENTALLY FROM THE PHYSICALLY ILL FOR TREATMENT AND MANAGEMENT

The treatment regimes of the Aesculapian temples do not appear to have distinguished between somatic and mental illnesses; all were treated in the same religiously oriented setting. The main treatment for both was suggestion through the use of ritual, though drugs such as helebore were also used with more or less specific intention to relieve particular symptoms. The first hospital specifically for the treatment of the mentally ill was founded in Jerusalem about 490 A.D. (Lewis, 1941), and the next millenium saw mental hospitals established all over Europe, Northern Africa, and the Near East.

Most of these early psychiatric "hospitals" were under the control of Catholic religious orders, at least until the Reformation. Zilboorg (1941) insists that these institutions did not deserve the name "hospital" at all, that they were merely places where the mentally ill were kept, not cared for or treated. Thus the early Bedlam, founded in 1247 in England, and Bicetre in France were "no more hospitals than a trench on a battlefield is a retreat of shelter and safety." He feels that the emergence of hospitals with therapeutic ideals did not occur until Pinel's and Chiarugi's reforms of the late 18th century. In any case, the Church-run hospitals were supported by the wealthy members of the community. These were usually also those with governmental authority. Thus it can be reasonably alleged that the support of the mentally ill in communities came from the state, though the immediate control of the institutions was private. The Reformation broke the Church's hold over the state, and the financial support of hospitals shifted to the emerging newer forms of government. Control of the institutions followed the source of financial support.

This change had already taken place by the time the American, British, French, and Spanish colonies were established. The first psychiatric hospital in the New World was established in 1566 in Mexico, the first in what is now the United States in Williamsburg, Virginia, in 1773. The first general hospital to admit "lunatics" was Pennsylvania Hospital in Philadelphia, in 1752 (Henry, 1941). The conditions of care in these and similar institutions was no better than those in contemporary European ones. Cruelty and neglect of the physical care of patients was the rule.

THE EMERGENCE OF "MORAL TREATMENT"

The reforms of Pinel led to the emergence of "moral treatment," largely under the influence of the Tuke family in England. The essence of this treatment scheme was that mental patients would respond normally to kindly, rational social approaches and that whether they did or not, they had a human status which demanded that they be so treated. A means of insuring moral treatment was that the caretakers of the ill should live closely with the patients, at best sharing the same table, as well as similar living quarters and cultural opportunities. These attractive principles were, however, very difficult to apply to large aggregations of patients because of financial stringencies that made impossible the employment of sufficient suitable personnel. The success of moral treatment led to the "cult of curability," a fascinating epidemic of conviction that practically all mental illnesses could be brought to recovery. This period was followed by one of disillusionment which, in part at least, contributed to another decline in the quality of care.

ADMINISTRATIVE PATTERNS IN THE UNITED STATES AND EUROPE

The care of the mentally ill in the American colonies, along with the chronically sick, retarded, criminals, and paupers was the responsibility of local, municipal, or county governments until the middle of the 19th century (Deutsch, 1937). These socially maladapted people were kept, usually miserably, in "poor houses" or in equally poor surroundings by their families. Diagnostic skills had improved, however, so that by the time Dorothea Dix instituted her reforms in the 1840s, it was possible to distinguish the mentally ill from other socially unsuccessful persons. Dix first turned her attention to the reform of the care of the mentally ill, but she was also active late in her career in prison reform (Marshall, 1937).

THE EMERGENCE OF THE STATE HOSPITAL IN THE UNITED STATES

The inclusion of the mentally ill with other groups of socially unsuccessful people also occurred in Europe. In England, for example, they were included in the administrative provisions of the "Poor Laws," and the mentally ill were housed with debtors and paupers, as so graphically described by Dickens in *The Pickwick Papers.* Distances were probably less of a problem in Europe than in the pioneer period in the United States; hence, the transfer of responsibility for the care of the mentally ill as they became identifiable shifted to central rather than local governments earlier there than was the case in the colonies.

Dix's main object was the establishment of hospitals for the mentally ill by state as contrasted to local governments. She saw that there were few specialists available to treat the many mentally ill. One of the principal reasons that the collection of patients in central hospitals was feasible in the middle 1800s was that roads, railroads, and steamships had developed and were present over most of the eastern United States. Dix's goal was to collect the patients in one place so that the specialist could treat them efficiently. In reaching this goal, she was magnificently successful. Neither she nor her supporters can be blamed for not being able to foresee that amassing large numbers of patients in hospitals would lead to the neglect of the individual needs of patients, or that it would later be found that care near the home was more desirable than care in a distant hospital.

WW I AND II: THEIR EFFECT ON MENTAL HEALTH ATTITUDES

World War I brought an acute recognition of the extent of mental and physical illness and mental deficiency in the young male population. The proportion of men incapable of becoming useful soldiers upon arrival in France was so large that Pershing protested and asked that the flow be stopped (Menninger, 1948). The deficiencies in the draftees were thought mainly to be related to poor care in infancy and childhood. This conclusion led to the development of nursery schools as a prophylactic institution in England, a movement that spread over the world.

It was also a factor leading to the establishment of the Children's Bureau of the U.S. Government in 1912 (Rosen, 1958).

In World War II, preenlistment physical and mental examinations were intensified and reduced the proportion of initial misfits, but breakdown under combat conditions, called "shell shock" in World War I and "combat exhaustion" in World War II, removed many soldiers from the fighting lines and occupied a considerable proportion of the military medical services (Menninger, 1948). Prophylaxis against these conditions was introduced in the form of intermittent relief from combat conditions and through morale building, educational efforts, and the training of officers in leadership technics. New methods of treatment were introduced and tested. One of the major principles that evolved during the war and that had great influence in later civilian developments was "treatment within the sound of the guns," that is, treatment in the situation where the stress was occurring and involving feelings of responsibility to others close to the individual and using their support in treatment. It is believed that this concept has been the source of much of the development of community psychiatry since World War II.

THE CRISIS IN U.S. PSYCHIATRIC HOSPITALIZATION

During World War II, military demands depleted personnel in the state psychiatric hospitals and led to the neglect of their buildings to such an extent that most of them were in a very poor state by the end of the war. Conditions were so bad that they led to a series of exposés revealing the enormous need for improvement (Wallace, 1949). The financial load of the construction of buildings and improvement of care was carried largely by the states; the federal government assiduously avoided becoming involved in the enormous funding problems involved in the care of the chronically mentally ill.

THE CITIZENS' MENTAL HEALTH MOVEMENT

As already noted, the care of the mentally ill has, almost throughout history, been deplorable. The miserable conditions of patients in jails or in areas provided by patients' families attracted the sympathy of citizens in Europe and were also the stimulus for Dorothea Dix and the many people she mobilized in her campaigns to better their situation. This citizen concern was organized in the United States by Clifford Beers. Himself a recovered patient, Beers wrote his influential book, *A Mind that Found Itself,* in 1908, and in 1909 organized the National Committee for Mental Hygiene. Its directing board included many of the illustrious psychiatrists of the country, such as Adolf Meyer; medical and public health leaders, such as William Welch and C.E.A. Winslow; and influential politicians and citizens. The movement grew gradually, establishing chapters in many states and municipalities and eventually internationally, as the World Federation for Mental Health. It not only was influential in the formation of public policy on the care of the mentally ill but also in the development of child guidance clinics and the emergence of the specialty of child psychiatry. It also stimulated research in mental illnesses, both by raising funds for this purpose and organizing professional advisory groups to plan and supervise them.

This group was deeply concerned about the situation of the system for the care of the mentally ill during and following World War II and was highly influential in obtaining the passage of the Mental Health Act of 1946.

THE DEVELOPMENT OF OUTPATIENT TREATMENT AND THE 1946 MENTAL HEALTH ACT

The federal government in the United States was induced to act in an entirely new direction designed to improve care outside hospitals and provide a prophylaxis against the need for hospitalization through early treatment in the community. The result was the National Mental Health Act of 1946, which had three stated goals: (1) the financing of education for psychiatrists, psychologists, psychiatric social workers, and psychiatric and mental health/public health nurses; (2) the financing of psychiatric and mental health research; and (3) providing incentive funds to the states for the establishment of mental health clinics.[1] The act also provided for a central administrative unit, the National Institute of Mental Health, and for a research and service center operated by the NIMH (PL79-487).

The National Institute of Mental Health grew from earlier efforts within the U.S. Public Health Service which, as early as 1920, had financed some mental health demonstration and outpatient services (Lemkau, 1955). Subsequent developments are reviewed by Ozarin (Chapter 2, this volume).

THE HISTORY OF PUBLIC HEALTH CONCEPTS AND ADMINISTRATIVE SCHEMES: THE MANAGEMENT OF PRESUMED ETIOLOGIES OF EPIDEMICS

Theories of the pathogenesis of disease have implicated etiologies arising from the environment since earliest recorded history. This probably was associated with the fact that the Greek, Roman, and Northern African populations suffered from endemic malaria and recognized that swamp waters, wind direction, and terrestrial altitude had something to do with the prevalence of recurrent bouts of chills and fever, though the intermediate host, the mosquito, was not recognized until much later. It was also recognized that filth and excrement were related to disease, so that cities developed methods of disposition that required an administrative system for their operation. It was further understood that disease and impure water were related, and that ample supplies of clean water helped keep filth and consequent epidemics under control. In order to provide clean streets, clean water, and proper sewage disposal, societies established various types of public authorities to administer the necessary programs.

Similarly, public authorities were involved in the disposition of dead bodies. It was recognized early that diseases were spread through commerce. One of the earliest public health measures, instituted first in Venice in 1127, was the isolation of newly arrived ships until it could be certain that no epidemic diseases were present in the crews. At one time this isolation lasted for 40 days, giving rise to the term "quarantine." It was also recognized early that some diseases were related to occupations such as mining, smelting metals, and, for a period, cider-making in which lead pipes were used.

With the emergence of the concept that many diseases were caused by germs, civil authorities were merged into departments of sanitary or medical police to ensure street cleanliness, clean water supplies, and reasonable disposal of sewage. These became the core of what were later public health services. The concept of the involvement of the environment in the causation of waves of disease in populations was embodied in the term "epidemic constitution."

PUBLIC HEALTH SERVICES AND THE CARE OF THE SICK

Even before the contagious and environmental sources of disease were realized, governments were also concerned with the care of the sick, particularly the poor of the community who were ill and could not pay for medical care. Early cities appointed physicians paid from public funds to care for the sick. As noted earlier, there was at first no distinction between mental and somatic illnesses, though later there was much argument as to whether the mentally ill were to be treated by philosophers or priests, as contrasted to physicians. In addition to these, however, there were the surgeons, usually of considerably less prestige, who set bones, "cut for (urinary) stone," and tended to military and other wounds. These three healing groups eventually merged into a single profession, medicine, but traces remain in the specialties of psychiatry, internal medicine, and surgery.

The function of medical services to particular groups in the population also became the responsibility of public health services. The U.S. Public Health Service grew out of the establishment by the government of special facilities for the care of merchant seamen. In the last few decades, however, the trend to combine multiple services such as water supply, sewage and waste disposal, and the care of the sick into public health services appears to be changing, particularly in the United States; water supply has become a function of civil engineering, and protection against occupational hazards is now a specialized field often not closely allied with other health services. The medical care of the poor is financed by administrative rather than medical organizations, with the medical function largely restricted to the provision of direct services in or out of a hospital.[2]

THE VIEWPOINTS OF THE PROFESSIONS OF MEDICINE AND PUBLIC HEALTH

The *Weltanschauungen,* or views of the world, of the professions of public health and of medicine are historically quite different. This is the case even though it is also recognized that the leaders in both areas have been men educated as physicians, though not exclusively so in either field. The barber-surgeons were not educated as medical men, and Pasteur, who made enormous contributions to both medicine and public health, was a chemist. Nevertheless, the generalization holds that the medical profession is preeminently concerned with the therapy of individuals who are sick and with preventing sickness in individuals. The specialty of public health finds its concerns with the health of populations, the reduction of the load of disease a population carries, and with devising methods with which the load of illness may be reduced through preventive and therapeutic means. The prime task that medicine takes upon itself is the care of the individual; the prime task of public health specialties is the reduction of the load of illness on a population.

This difference in primary interest, which of course could not have been defined clearly in early medical history, carries with it somewhat contrasting approaches to the problems of the etiology of disease. Practitioners of medicine are likely to look for the etiology of diseases within the individual being treated. Their interest will be primarily diagnostic and therapeutic, and only secondarily involved in ways to keep the next case from occurring. Thus, although they recognize that infection or poisoning must come from the environment, they are likely to be more interested in what is happening to the patient than in the source of the infection or poison. This attitude, certainly the ideal for individual care, has been severely criticized as the "medical model," implying that it is too individually rather than socially oriented, and that it looks too much for etiological factors "within the skin" of the patient rather than in societal and interindividual, etiological sources.

The scope of possible etiologies falling within the scope of the public health specialist touches a much wider segment of "natural philosophy," to use a term once applied to all scientific endeavor. The ancient term, "epidemic constitution," for example, included factors such as the "miasma" arising from filth, the altitude above sea level, the direction of the wind, and the nutritional, financial, and general health status of the population in its confusing definition. As already noted, such concerns made public health an integral part of government very early in history, a situation which has persisted since. Leighton recognized the importance of the inclusive view of etiologies in mental illnesses by using a quote from Virchow, who lived from 1821-1902, in her epidemiological study of mental illnesses, *The Character of Danger.* The need to consider a wide range of etiological agents and situations in considering mental illnesses tends to pull psychiatry away from general medical practice and toward the broader public health stand, in that societal and interpersonal factors are more often considered as parts of an etiological complex.

MENTAL HEALTH AND ITS PUBLIC HEALTH AND MEDICAL CARE INTERRELATIONSHIPS

Mental illnesses and disorders, at least at the present state of knowledge, require the broad view of etiology historically espoused by public health. The treatment of individual patients, however, often requires intensive attention to the personal, individual experiences of the patient. This has made practitioners of psychiatry one of the groups most insistent upon medical confidentiality. Perhaps it has also contributed to the relative underdevelopment of the epidemiology of mental illnesses as compared to infectious, cardiovascular, or oncological disease. The ancient mysteries surrounding the priests who once claimed the care of the mentally ill still seems to invite a touch-me-not attitude toward the use of personal data in the study of mental illnesses and disorders. The mental health profession appears thus to be attracted by the breadth of public health etiologic concepts but repelled by the necessity to make facts available for epidemiologic study.

To a considerable extent, a similar situation exists in the relationship of practitioners of psychiatry to practitioners of other medical specialties. Psychiatrists and other mental health specialists express the hope that they may be incorporated and may incorporate themselves more fully into the field of medical practice and public health. On the other hand, it seems they often demand separate treatment. Thus, the National Institute for Mental Health has repeatedly resisted full integration into the organization of the National Institutes of Health. I recall that the National Mental Health Advisory Council, of which I was then a member, refused to endorse the Woolford Report (NIH Study Committee, 1965), which recommended an amalgamation of services, nor did it support a replication of a planning activity already completed by the states for mental health facilities by the rest of health services (PL81-749). Usually such separatist actions have been taken in support of the contention that the amalgamation of mental health with other public health services would result in reduced visibility of the mental health field with a consequent reduction of funding for it. I suspect that the conflict between the evaluation of social etiologies and the insistence on confidentiality are also of importance.

Nor has public health embraced mental health efforts enthusiastically. The American Public Health Association has only included a mental health section for the last 25 years. One historical reason that public health administrations have been reluctant to incorporate mental health activities has been the enormous financial load of the traditional mental hospital system; the fear was that the "tail" of mental hospital financing would wag the "dog," i.e., the other public health services (Lemkau, 1955). This situation has changed, however. Public health authorities in many states have expanded from prevention, consultation, and laboratory services to include, first, tuberculosis hospitalization and later, chronic disease institutionalization and the support of medical care for the indigent. On the other hand, mental hospitals have decreased their populations (though not their costs) considerably, making the financial argument less tenable.

With the expansion of mental health services at the local community level by the federal government, beginning with the 1946 Mental Health Act and extended by the 1963 Mental Health Centers Act and the 1980 Mental Health Systems Act,[3] mental health had need of an organizational base at the local rather than the state level. The catchment area, under the 1963

Act, was to include 75,000 to 200,000 persons. In urban areas there were likely to be enough catchment area units to justify separate administrative organizations for coordinating the activities of the several centers. In rural areas, however, catchment areas were likely to include rather large geographic areas—in at least one case, 20 counties. In this situation, housing of the center activities and the administration of the program could not justify a separate administration. In rural situations, the mental health operations, in at least some states, more or less fell back to the pre-Dorothea Dix status of county administration, but not usually to the local public health administrative agency. In other states, however, the administration of local mental health operations remained a state responsibility of the mental health authority, which was itself often a part of a larger Human Resources state administrative unit.

SUMMARY AND FORECAST

In earlier history, mental as well as all other types of illness common to etiologies less obvious than those of wounds or broken bones were believed to be of supernatural origin. As time passed, more specific etiological factors appeared for specific types of illnesses. Those illnesses with exclusively mental symptomatology were more resistant to etiological and pathological explication and appear to have remained longer in the realm of supernatural etiology than other types of illnesses. Gradually, the concept of a multifactorial etiology of these (and other) diseases evolved, supplanting the notion of a supernatural etiology. This brought the etiological theories of psychiatry close to the theories of causation needed to confront public health issues. On the other hand, treatment remained intensely individual, so that comparative epidemiologic study was difficult. These problems have tended to keep mental health efforts isolated both from the general practice of medicine and from full inclusion in public health administrative operations; practical fiscal matters also tended to keep the fields apart.

What does the future hold? It has become obvious in the 20th century that no disease or illness is the result of a single etiological factor. The director of a tuberculosis hospital once told me that none of his patients ever got sick without having undergone some sort of family stress. It has been recognized since the earliest recorded history that the poor suffer more illness than the better-off in the population. In the future, knowledge of the multifactorial causation of disease and disorder will receive more recognition. As it does, the so-called "medical model" will recognize more frankly and fully the legitimacy of the broad scope of psychiatric and public health etiologic thinking.

With the appearance of nudity and sexual intercourse in movies, and with discussion of abortion, contraception, and teenage pregnancy in all the media, it appears that there may be better opportunities for the epidemiological analysis of personal, interpersonal, and societal etiologic factors for mental illnesses and disorders in the future. Medical confidentiality may be less of a hindrance to scientific analysis of etiologic situations than it has been in the past.

The advances in neuropathology and neurophysiology of the last few decades will probably simplify etiological concepts considerably. The mechanism by which the nervous system somehow produces somatic feelings of discomfort in situations of psychological stress may become clearer and more specific, so that more direct and specific measures to relieve stress, improve its personal management, or interrupt the symptom-producing process are possible and disease or disorder prevented. Finally, health services needed by the population and that society decides are the responsibility of government may be administered by a single agency, at least at the local governmental level.

Notes

1. Although the 1946 Mental Health Act did not specify that outpatient treatment was to be promoted, the language ("and assisting states in the use of the most effective methods of prevention, diagnosis and treatment of psychiatric disorders") was interpreted so that no funds could be used for the support of patients already in mental hospitals. There was thus an invitation to the states to use the money to increase services outside hospitals.

2. The essence of this brief survey of the history of public health is from Rosen (1941) and from courses in the history of public health taught by Oswei Temkin. The abbreviation presented here includes interpretations that are, however, the author's. Rosen's coverage and the original sources are strongly recommended for further reading in the history of public health.

3. The changes and proposed changes in the federal funding of mental health services, involving to a considerable but not uniform extent changes in funding from direct grants to facilities to block grants to states, together with uncertainties about the federal budget, make it impossible at the time this is written to delinate how and to what extent the Mental Health Systems Act will eventually operate. See Ozarin (Chapter 2, this volume) and Wagenfeld and Jacobs (Chapter 3, this volume) for more on this.

References

BEERS, C. W. *A mind that found itself: An autobiography.* New York: Longmans, Green, 1908.

DEUTSCH, A. *The mentally ill in America.* New York: Doubleday, 1937.

HENRY, G. W. Quoted in G. Zilboorg, *A history of medical psychology.* New York: W. W. Norton, 1941.

LEMKAU, P. V. *Mental hygiene in public health.* New York: McGraw-Hill, 1955.

LEWIS, N.D.C. *A short history of psychiatric achievement.* New York: W. W. Norton, 1941.

MARSHALL, H. *Dorothea Dix: Forgotten samaritan.* Chapel Hill: University of North Carolina Press, 1937.

MENNINGER, W. *Psychiatrist for a troubled world.* New York: MacMillan, 1948.

NIH Study Committee. *Biomedical science and its administration: A study of the National Institutes of Health.* Report to the President, February 1965. Washington, DC: Government Printing Office.

ROSEN, G. *A history of public health.* New York: M.D., 1958.

WALLACE, W. *Maryland's shame.* Baltimore: The Sunpapers, 1949.

ZILBOORG, G. *A history of medical psychology.* New York: W. W. Norton, 1941.

Chapter 2

MENTAL HEALTH IN PUBLIC HEALTH
The Federal Perspective

LUCY D. OZARIN

THE BEGINNING

The last quarter-century has seen a flowering of interest in joining public health and mental health, but the story begins earlier. While the practice of public health gained strength and effectiveness during the latter part of the last century and the earlier years of this century, psychiatry and mental health largely remained in a world apart, sequestered in the remote mental hospitals of those days. The Federal Immigration Service was concerned about mental illness among immigrants, and several narcotic "farms" had been established, but not until 1930 did the renamed Narcotics Division of the U.S. Public Health Service become the Division of Mental Hygiene. Under the directorship of Dr. Lawrence Kolb, Sr. (1938-1944) arose the concept of a National Neuropsychiatric Institute, which came into being in Public Law 79-487, July 3, 1946, known as the National Mental Health Act. Dr. Robert H. Felix had followed Kolb in the director's job in 1944, and he became director of the newly created National Institute of Mental Health (NIMH).

The NIMH was unique in that the Mental Health Act authorized a tripartite program to include research and research training, training in mental health disciplines through academic settings, and the improvement of community-based mental health services, demonstrations, and training of personnel for state and local health work. Brand and Sapir (1964) note that the act was drafted in the tradition of limited federal action in curative medicine. From this beginning, public health, mental health, and the NIMH have been intertwined. It is no accident that the first three directors had all received formal public health training (1949-1979).

The disbursing of funds by the NIMH for community mental health programs was not unique, since the Public Health Service had already been providing categorical grants-in-aid to public health departments for control and prevention programs in cancer, tuberculosis, venereal disease, and other areas of significance to public health (Public Health Services Act, Sec. 202, PL78-410). The Mental Health Act stated that community funds were for the purpose of developing and assisting states in the use of the most effective methods of prevention, diagnosis, and treatment of psychiatric disorders. Since the categorical grants-in-aid were paid to the State Health Authority, the act defined the term State Mental Health Authority to "mean the State Health Authority except that in the case of any State in which there is a single State agency, other than the State Health Authority, charged with the responsibility for administering the mental health program of the State, it means such other State agency." A General Circular issued on March 23, 1949 by the Federal Security Agency (predecessor of DHEW) on the organization of the NIMH states: "The Institute shall collaborate with the Bureau of State Services to develop such community mental health services in reasonable conformity with patterns and organizations of the various PHS programs now in operation."

In 1949, when the NIMH came into existence, every state was operating one or more mental hospitals, but only a few of the larger states had state-level mental hygiene departments with interests in community programs. In 1946, only 22 states had a mental health program other than mental hospitals. State hospitals often operated under the aegis of various boards or other state-level agencies. Thus, the State Health Department in many states became the Mental Health Authority. This was a new role, and often staff with little or no mental health preparation were appointed to develop a program. The small categorical grant was used in various ways: for mental health education, to assist local groups to start an outpatient psychiatric clinic, or to provide mental health input to other health department programs, such as maternal and child health. Meanwhile, many state hospitals had developed outpatient and posthospital followup programs.

The disadvantages of a state health department or other agency became obvious through the 1950s when joint planning and coordinated efforts were not always followed. Many states eventually transferred the State Mental Health Authority to the state-level department that also operated the mental hospitals program.

It is of interest to note that with the designation of state health departments as the Mental Health Authority in conformance with the Mental Health Act, the effort was made to orient public health officers about mental health. In 1948, a two-week conference was held in California, bringing together a number of these officers with mental health experts to discuss the relatedness of public health and mental health. The report of the conference was published under the title *Public Health is People* (1950).

During the 1950, with their ties to public health departments, many mental health programs concentrated their efforts on primary and secondary prevention, including early treatment in some places. In terms of primary prevention, mental health education materials were produced and distributed with an emphasis on child rearing and development. These efforts suffered because the conceptual and substantive bases for preventing mental disorders, in contrast to infectious disease, were quite limited. The conceptual basis for preventive efforts was broadened later with the publication of the Midtown Manhattan and Stirling County studies (Srole et al., 1962; Leighton & Leighton, 1954). These epidemiological investigations found high levels of mental disorder in the general population and postulated an etiological link between stress and disorder.

The relationship of social problems to mental health had been noted on the federal level as early as 1950. One NIMH publication states: "Many social problems are closely related to mental ill health, especially crime, delinquency, divorce, and alcoholism" (Federal Security Agency, 1950). Later, Felix (1964) was to quote Adolph Meyers's belief that the domain of psychiatry is the behavior of the entire man as he reacts to the stresses of his environment.

Secondary prevention efforts were directed at early identification and treatment of those with mental and emotional problems and disorders. Community outpatient clinics were the major means. In the early 1920s, a group of demonstration child guidance clinics had been established, and gradually through the 1930s a small number of adult psychiatric clinics also came into being. By 1947, an estimated 600 outpatient clinics existed. In 1948 the NIMH established an outpatient clinic in Prince Georges County, Maryland, under the direction of Mabel Ross, M.D., as a demonstration in community mental health which later took on a research focus. The original goal was to test the application of public health methods in the operation of a community mental health program. By 1955, about 1300 outpatient clinics had been established.

Tertiary prevention, the prevention and amelioration of disability, was left entirely within the domain of the mental hospitals. In the 1970s, amendments to the Rehabilitation and Developmental Disabilities legislation (PL73-112, 1973 and following years) specifically mentioned the mentally ill to be included within the purview of rehabilitation programs.

Efforts in tertiary prevention were also supported by congressional action in amending the Public Health Services Act in 1956 (Title V) to fund investigations, experiments, and research looking toward improved diagnosis, care, treatment, and rehabilitation of the mentally ill. A wide variety of activities were supported, particularly in the aftercare and rehabilitation activities directed toward previously hospitalized patients. Between 1958 and 1964, 559 projects were funded. In 1964, Congress added an item in the NIMH budget to support projects solely in public mental hospitals for the improvement of patient care. These projects truly fell within the realm of tertiary prevention. In the first five years of the Hospital Improvement Program (HIP), over 120,000 patients were involved in a large number of projects dealing with preparing chronic patients to leave the mental hospital. The HIP program was later phased into the current Community Support Program for chronic patients living in community settings.

COMMUNITY MENTAL HEALTH ACTS

The states also enacted community mental health legislation beginning in 1954. In that year, New York passed the first community mental health act to provide financial support for local mental health activities. Hunt and Forstenzer (1957) and Forstenzer and Hunt (1958) recount the background of the act and its early development. Lemkau (1957), commenting on the New York act, wrote: "The very existence of the Act constitutes official recognition of the fact that mental health is a public health problem."

Similar legislation was passed in California and Minnesota in 1957 and, soon after, in New Jersey (Ozarin, 1962). Other state legislative actions began to provide funds for community mental health. In 1957, a Georgia law provided funds for the care of psychiatric patients in general hospitals. Some state legislation required the establishment of local mental health boards (New York, 1954); others provided support directly to providers (Connecticut, 1957). The state mental health central offices promulgated rules and regulations to implement the legislation, provided technical assistance, and were responsible for administering the acts.

By 1969, 34 states had passed community mental health acts, and practically all state legislatures now budget funds for local community mental health activities (see Wagenfeld and Jacobs, Chapter 3, this volume).

TRAINING PROGRAMS

With the growing thrust to establish local services, increasing numbers of trained personnel were needed. The National Mental

Health Act had authorized support for training, and by 1970 about 30 percent of the NIMH annual budget was directed toward academic and other training institutions for accredited training in psychiatry, psychology, social service, psychiatric and mental health nursing, other social sciences, and research training. This percentage has now decreased by half. The NIMH also provided funds to medical schools to foster teaching about human development, mental health, and psychiatry to undergraduate medical students in an effort to spread mental health principles to all pertinent medical fields.

In 1948, mental health manpower included 4,500 psychiatrists, 1,500 psychologists, 1,000 psychiatric social workers, and 5,500 nurses working in mental hospitals. By 1969, these figures had increased to 23,500 psychiatrists, 29,000 psychologists, 50,000 social workers (not all working in mental health settings), and 31,000 nurses working in hospital and community mental health settings. Special graduate nursing programs in mental health had been established at the Columbia and Johns Hopkins public health schools. At the present time, total manpower includes approximately 30,000 psychiatrists, 27,000 psychologists with Ph.D.s (additional master's-level psychologists have been trained), a total of 53,000 registered nurses working in psychiatric and mental health settings, 6,000 nurses with master's degrees in mental health/psychiatric nursing, and 80,000 master's-level social workers, of whom about 25,000 work in mental health settings (see Penn, Chapter 7, this volume and Rieman, Chapter 8, this volume). The workers and their training institutions have not in every case received NIMH support, although the majority of training sites have received assistance. The Veterans Administration has supported training for the four core disciplines—psychiatry, psychology, social work, and psychiatric nursing—since World War II.

Nor was the role of the nonpsychiatric physician neglected. Beginning in 1959, a series of grants was made to provide psychiatric knowledge to nonpsychiatrists to assist them in identifying mental disorders among their patients, to deal with those disorders within their capability, and to refer to psychiatrists or psychiatric clinics as necessary. Between 1959 and 1968, more than 10,000 physicians had participated in this type of training (Webster & Ozarin, 1968). The role of the general practitioner in mental health is receiving increasing attention at present. Another NIMH program supported general practitioners who were entering psychiatric residency training. Note should also be taken that NIMH funds supported mental health training in schools of public health from 1947 until the early 1970s.

The early years of mental health programs (apart from mental hospitals) were firmly based and rooted in public health. But a variety of forces came into play to separate them in the 1950s. World War II had directed attention to mental disability, both because of large numbers of rejectees for military service and the toll of psychiatric disorders in the military forces. Also, because of wartime experiences and an increasing patient load in Veteran Administration facilities, psychiatric and mental health-related training was sought and encouraged, and an increasing number of mental health professionals, especially psychiatrists, entered private practice. As a result, the need arose for psychiatric hospital beds in general hospitals to serve the patients of a growing cadre of privately practicing mental health professionals that now includes social workers, psychologists, and mental health and psychiatric nurses. However, many private practitioners, in addition to their individual practices, work part-time in community mental health and social agencies in the public domain.

Public interest in mental health after World War II led to investigations into and publicity about conditions in public mental hospitals that in many cases were appalling in their overcrowding, lack of staff, and inadequate physical facilities. As a result of the publicity and the realization by psychiatric and mental health leaders (NIMH, National Association of Mental Health, and professional organizations) that the time was ripe to seek alternatives to public mental hospitals as the major locus of mental health treatment, Congress was importuned to pass the Mental Health Study Act (PL84-182) in 1955, which provided funds to NIMH to study the national needs and resources in mental health. The Commission on Mental Health and Illness was formed by 36 participating organizations that hired a staff under the directorship of Dr. Jack Ewalt. The commission and its staff (under NIMH contract) carried out a number of studies, and on December 31, 1960 presented its report, *Action for Mental Health,* to the President and Congress.

The commission's recommendations generally paralleled the congressional directives expressed in the Mental Health Act of 1947, namely, more research into the causes of mental illness, more mental health manpower through augmented training programs, and the establishment of community programs as an alternative to large custodial mental hospitals. Also included were recommendations on care for chronic mental patients and public information programs.

This chapter will not recount the developments following the Joint Commission report. In 1963, a presidential message on Mental Retardation and Mental Illness was sent to Congress, and passage of the Community Mental Health Centers Act followed (see Wagenfeld & Jacobs, Chapter 3, this volume). Congress has given consistent and continuous support to community mental health programs, enlarging the scope of the original act in its subsequent amendments and culminating in the Mental Health Systems Act of 1980, which superseded the earlier legislation. The MHSA became inoperative before its implementation through administrative action replacing it with a single mental health alcohol and drug abuse block grant to states in 1981 (Omnibus Reconciliation Act of 1981, PL97-75).

Community mental health programs have achieved a measure of success in making services available to more than half the people in this country through almost 800 federally assisted CMHCs. In addition, an array of private and public facilities and practitioners also provide mental health services. In 1955, three-fourths of psychiatric episodes occurred in mental hospitals. Currently, three-fourths of such episodes occur in nonresidential settings. Twenty years ago, the major diagnoses of people seen in mental health facilities were psychoses. These are in the minority now, while diagnoses of depression, alcohol and drug abuse, maladjustment, and personality disorders have increased. In the past, one-third of all admissions to mental hospitals related to older people with disorders of the senium; today, only about 10 percent are so related, albeit with a nursing home population of a million and estimates that more than half of this population have diagnosable mental conditions.

Developments in health insurance and other forms of third-party payers have led to the insured seeking private care. Those who seek public care or care through organized facilities are usually the poor without other resources, those who live in remote areas without private mental health practitioners, or those who experience an acute psychiatric emergency.

Comprehensive community mental health programs, as exemplified by the CMHC program, have embodied public health principles. They require a population base, a program directed at a defined geographic service area. They require a needs assessment of the population to be served so that programs can be directed to priority needs and to identify noxious environmental factors. They seek to coordinate community resources, inject mental health principles into the work of people-serving agencies through consultation and training, and to provide mental health education and information to the public. While community programs use public health principles, though often not planfully, relationships with organized public health agencies are limited, often to public health nurses.

The work of the pioneers in mental health/public health has taken root, and public health principles are accepted as an integral part of organized mental health programs. In 1962, the Program Area Committee on Mental Health of the APHA published a monograph titled *Mental Disorders: A Guide to Control Methods.* It was thought that the guide might serve a function similar to the APHA's manual on *Control of Communicable Diseases in Man.* The guide presented an estimate of existing tools for modifying the amount of mental disorder in a population. The monograph noted that estimates are needed to answer such questions as: What can be done through organized health programs by governments and voluntary agencies and through community action to reduce the size of the burden created by mental disorders? What can be done to shorten the duration of mental disorders that have already occurred? and What can be done to reduce the amount of disability and distress caused by unpreventable or nonterminable disorders?

The guide considered various mental disorders of known and unknown etiology and proposed preventive measures, including support in times of stress, prevention of maternal deprivation, improvement in child rearing practices, prenatal care, and genetic counseling. Other topics covered data collection and analyses for program planning and evaluation, research methods, and implications for training.

In 1975, another publication, this one titled *Mental Health: The Public Health Challenge,* was issued by the APHA. This was a project begun in 1972 by the Mental Health Section. The introduction states: "The changing panorama of mental health services, training, and research in relation to public health and individual well being is a national challenge. . . . There now exists an opportunity to make important changes in how services are delivered and resources used." The monograph discusses the changes, saying: "Much of the future of mental health and mental retardation planning and administration and quality assurance will be in the hands of the States. It is they, rather than the Federal government who have the responsibility of carrying out the service programs." The introduction points out the need for linking mental health services with other health- and social service-related systems and discusses standard setting, quality assurance, third-party payer provisions, and multiple-source funding, all important for planning and implementation. Systems of care are emphasized. The aim of the volume is to provide stimulus and guidelines to improve mental health systems and encourage new explorations in using mental health skills in the interest of personal and family growth and on significant social issues, but without claiming omnipotence in tangential areas.

The two APHA mental health publications indicate the shift that occurred between 1962-1975 from a concentration on illness and disorder to the inclusion of prevention and social environmental factors as they impinge on communities and individuals. Felix (1964) wrote: "We are concerned with a framework of service that admits to no separation of prevention, treatment and rehabilitation."

Dr. Stanley Yolles (1965), whose directorship of the NIMH coincided with the Civil Rights movement and other activities of the late 1960s, emphasized this approach, saying: "Unresolved major social problems may be the unsanitary breeding grounds for chronic mental stress." Later, Yolles (1969) wrote:

"A CMHC has two primary missions; one is to provide treatment to any person (in need). . . . The second is to improve the quality of life for people in a community through a wide variety of avenues including the improvement of the physical environment and the educational and cultural opportunities of whole communities."

Dr. Bertram Brown (1971), third director of the NIMH, speaking on the same theme, said the challenge is to provide humane and effective care to the mentally ill, to determine the causes of mental and emotional breakdown, and to promote mental health, and that "the objective is and must be that every child and person have a chance to fulfill his full potential as a creative, productive, human being. . . . It is little wonder that the mental health movement began in this country as a social issue as well as an issue of public health. . . . We are still closely involved with the matters of social and public policy."

In the final analysis, legislators, other policymakers, and third-party payers may be the decision makers who will determine the nature of mental health and what services they are willing to pay for. For the present, we know that the toll of mental dysfunction is great enough to constitute a public health problem, we are accumulating an epidemiologic data base to serve as a foundation to plan programs, and we have found some techniques that can be used effectively in primary, secondary, and tertiary prevention in both behavioral and social dysfunction.

TOWARD THE FUTURE

In the study cited earlier, Yolles (1969: 21) projected the nature of community mental health services in 1980. He wrote: "There is evidence that community psychiatry is well on its way to provision of effective help for individuals; development of new trends in community action will be one of the major trends of the next decade. The NIMH is expanding its support of programs that will be helpful to the poor and socially disadvantaged and related to their needs. . . . The community mental health center is the best model available for services demanded by the poor." Yolles also mentions training for professionals to work with all races, social and economic groups, and research programs to continue to supply new knowledge and innovations. "The objective of the mental health program in the U.S. is to bring all pertinent resources to bear to discover better physical and social structures for modern living . . . to include attempts to examine the human condition and human behavior in their total living context" (Yolles, 1969: 22). Noted also are the emergence of new social structures and new fields of scientific activity, including behavior genetics, ethnomedicine, urbanology, and others.

Yolles's projections for 1980 have been realized only in part. The Mental Health Systems Act (PL96-398) embodied some aspects, but even before its implementation it was superseded by the block grant mechanism that places full responsibility and authority for mental health programs within each state. In the past, states have been supportive of comprehensive community mental health programs as evidenced by their support for non-profit and public community mental health centers, which in most states receive 30-40 percent of their total operating expenses from state governments. However, the political and fiscal realities of 1982, with reduced budgets, are bound to lead to some curtailment of activities. The State Mental Health Authority will have to negotiate with the state funding agency for its fair share of the federal mental health, alcohol and drug abuse block grant.

The role of the federal government in relation to service delivery would then become that of data collection and analyses, technical assistance to state and local agencies and other groups, and research to produce new knowledge. It is not clear how the training of mental health manpower will be funded. Leadership and overall direction of mental health programs at the federal level will need to continue, since only at that level is it possible to accumulate the nationwide information for those tasks. Local agencies will deliver service in accordance with state guidelines and standards, but what will be the form and pattern of those services? Funding will determine that answer.

The literature contains numerous writings about the role of the state hospital of the future (Talbott, 1978; Ahmed & Plog, 1976; Zusman, 1973; Rutman & Egan, 1975). Statements have been made about the closing of public mental hospitals, beginning with Dr. Harry Solomon in 1958. A small group of hospitals have closed as community services have become available (California, Massachusetts), but the total number of public mental hospitals shows little difference from 1946. In some states, the functions of the state hospitals have changed.[1] The state hospital perforce has had to accommodate its programs to the total community mental health program in the state. But as it has done historically, the state hospital is still filling the gaps in service and is still the major institution that cares for chronic and difficult psychiatric patients.

The movement of large numbers of chronic and handicapped patients from mental hospitals to community residence as a result of the availability of psychotrophic drugs and federal funding for their support (SSI, Medicaid, Medicare, Vocational Rehabilitation) has posed a major problem in that community services do not match their need. Also, both professional and public opinion is mounting that some of these expatients are better served by remaining in the hospital or in sheltered settings as intermediate care facilities. Recognition is growing, reinforced by mounting readmission rates (up to 75 percent), that some patients need continuing "asylum." Some thought is being given to establishing new types of care facilities for patients who do not fit into the already established range of housing opportunities: cooperative apartments, foster homes, and psychosocial rehabilitation facilities (DHHS, 1980).

There is no support for continuing the huge mental institutions of the past (at one time, Pilgrim State Hospital in New York housed 14,000 patients). Smaller state hospitals have appeared (the regional mental hospitals in Georgia range from about 200 to 400 beds). Many of the formerly large state hospitals are now drastically reduced in size. Hospital organization and administration as well as treatment programs change as size changes. But a hospital under state aegis presents problems, as Talbott (1980) has pointed out. The social ethos of the 1970s has led to increasing citizen involvement. Community mental health nonprofit agencies have citizen boards that serve as advocates for the agencies. An informed citizenry has long been an asset in mental health undertakings. The 1980s are also presenting a thrust away from federal regulation toward giving responsibility for mental health to states and down to community level. It is not clear how these social philosophies will result in services for the person who needs help. It is clear that less money will be available for community mental health, and that all avenues for assistance need exploration.

One promising avenue is through the providers of health care. Research has shown that over half of all patients seen by nonpsychiatrists have diagnosable mental conditions, and that only 20 percent of these cases are referred to mental health specialists (Regier et al., 1978). Many people do not recognize their symptoms as related to nonphysical conditions and visit physicians for help. Research has also shown that psychiatric interventions reduce the need for physical care (Locke et al., 1966). Demonstration has been carried out to shown the feasibility of providing mental health expertise in health care settings (Borus et al., 1979). It is likely that the future will see expansion of such efforts. However, health providers will require special training if they are to provide care for the more seriously mentally ill. It is likely that acutely psychotic patients will continue to be treated by psychiatrists and mental health personnel, but chronic patients who are shown to be high users of physical care could be treated by health care personnel who receive training, supervision, and consultation from mental health professionals.

A new problem is also being recognized (Pepper, 1981). New "young chronic patients," some of whom have never been in state hospitals, are growing in numbers. These people have different needs compared with the old chronic patients who spent many years in state hospitals. It is this group for whom new types of organizational structures may be needed: intermediate care, asylums, hostels, temporary shelters. The solution will depend on the availability of funding, research, and demonstration. For the present, the state hospital remains the major resource.

While we struggle to deal with the problems of mental illness and dysfunction, the push to find prevention for these problems continues. Research continues into infant and childhood development, family functioning, job stress, unemployment, marital stress, and aging. As findings are produced, they are fed into the fabric of life through our numerous social structures, schools, churches, workplaces, courts, recreation sites, and others. As is true in public health, where many preventive measures are carried out by nonhealth personnel (safe water, clean air), prevention of mental disorders will no doubt become part of everyday living.

EPILOGUE

There are no easy solutions to problems of mental illness and health. The social and political processes in our country will have as much to do with solutions as will mental health expertise. But there is certainty on one point: Treatment and care of the mentally ill and those troubled by mental problems is more available and more effective today than it has been at any time in the past 100 years. There is every reason to believe that it will be better in the years to come. We know some tasks to be done and more will unfold. If we remember basic public health philosophy and methods, our tasks will be easier.

Note

1. In California, the state hospital accepts only patients referred by the county mental health authorities after the patient has received evaluation and treatment and provides only inpatient care; in New York, some state hospitals (e.g., Harlem Valley) have become an integral part of the local scene.

References

AHMED, P. I., & PLOG, S. C. *State mental hospitals: What happens when they close.* New York: Plenum, 1976.

BELLAK, L., & BARTEN, H. H. (Eds.) *Progress in community mental health.* New York: Grune & Stratton, 1969.

BORUS, J., BURNS, B., JACOBSON, A., MACHT, L. B., MORRILL, R. G., & WILSON, E. M. *Coordinated mental health care in neighborhood health centers in mental health services in general health care.* Vol. 2. Washington, DC: National Academy of Science, Institute of Medicine, 1979.

BRAND, J. L., & SAPIR, P. *A historical perspective on the National Institute of Mental Health.* NIMH, 1964.

BROWN, B. S. *The once and future challenge.* National Institute of Mental Health's 25th Anniversary Conference, Washington, D.C., June 1971.

Commonwealth Fund. *Public health is people: An institute on mental health in public health held at Berkeley, California in 1948.* New York: Commonwealth Fund, 1950.

Department of Health and Human Services, Steering Committee on the Chronically Mentally Ill. *Toward a national plan for the chronically mentally ill.* Washington, DC: Public Health Service, 1980.

Federal Security Agency. *The National Mental Health Act and your community.* Washington, DC: Government Printing Office, Mental Health Series No. 3, 1950.

FELIX, R. H. *Report to the Congress, 1964.* Collected papers, National Institute of Mental Health, Washington, D.C., 1964.

FORSTENZER, H., & HUNT, R. C. The New York State Mental Health Services Act: Its origins and the first four years of development. *Psychiatric Quarterly Supplement,* 1958, *32,* 41-67.

HUNT, R. C., & FORESTENZER, H. The New York State Community Mental Health Services Act: Its birth and early development. *American Journal of Psychiatry,* 1957, *113,* 68-685.

LEIGHTON, A. H., & LEIGHTON, D. C. *My name is legion.* New York: Basic Books, 1954.

LEMKAU, P., FURMAN, S., FARBMAN, K., LAY, M., & BAILEY, M. The operation of the New York State Community Mental Health Services Act in New York City. *American Journal of Psychiatry,* 1957, *113,* 686-690.

LOCKE, B. Z., KRANTZ, G., & KRAMER, M. Psychiatric need and demand for a prepaid group practice program. *American Journal of Public Health,* 1966, *56,* 895-904.

OZARIN, L. Recent community mental health legislation: A brief review. *American Journal of Public Health,* 1962, *52.*

PEPPER, B., KIRSHNER, M., & RYGLEWICZ, H. The young adult chronic patient: Overview of a population. *Journal of Hospital and Community Psychiatry,* 1981, *32,* 463-469.

REGIER, D. A., GOLDBERG, I. D., & TAUBE, C. A. The de facto U.S. mental health services system. *Archives of General Psychiatry,* 1978, *35,* 685-693.

RUTMAN, I. D., & EGAN, K. L. *The future role of the state mental hospital.* Philadelphia: Horizon House Institute for Research and Development, 1975.

SOLOMON, H. The American Psychiatric Association in relation to American psychiatry. *American Journal of Psychiatry,* 1958, *115,* 1-9.

SROLE, L., LANGNER, T. S., MICHAEL, S. T., OPLER, M. K., & RENNIE, T.A.L. *Mental health in the metropolis.* New York: McGraw-Hill, 1962.

TALBOTT, J. *Death of the asylum: A critical study of state hospital management, services, and care.* New York: Grune & Stratton, 1978.

TALBOTT, J. *State hospitals, problems and potentials.* New York: Human Sciences Press, 1980.

WEBSTER, T. G., & OZARIN, L. D. Federal funds for continuing education in mental health programs. *Journal of Hospital and Community Psychiatry,* 1968, *19,* 47-52.

YOLLES, S. Integration of mental health planning into public health planning. Paper presented at Caribbean seminar in mental health, Kingston, Jamaica, September 1965.

YOLLES, S. *Past, present and 1980: Trend projections in community mental health,* Vol. I, 1969.

ZUSMAN, J. (Ed.) *The future role of the state hospital.* Buffalo: State University of New York, 1973.

Chapter 3

THE COMMUNITY MENTAL HEALTH MOVEMENT
Its Origins and Growth

MORTON O. WAGENFELD and JUDITH H. JACOBS

The two previous chapters in this section have touched on community mental health in the context of discussing the development of public mental health. Other chapters in this volume consider manpower and training issues as a result of the rapid expansion of community mental health centers. Since community mental health has been variously described as the "Third Psychiatric Revolution" (Bellak, 1964) and the "Belief System of the '60s" (Schulberg & Baker, 1969), it is necessary that any volume on public mental health focus directly on the origins, growth, current state, and probable future of community mental health centers (CMHCs) and the community mental health movement. In doing so, we will be drawing insights and data from a variety of sources.

From a sociological perspective, the community mental health movement exhibits all of the characteristics of a social movement: leaders, followers, an ideology and program, and

---

Authors' Note: We are grateful to Fred Spaner for sharing with us some of his insights on the development of the CMHC legislation. This chapter was prepared in a private capacity. The opinions or views expressed are those of the authors and do not necessarily reflect the official policy of the National Institute of Mental Health.

some bureaucratic structure (Blumer, 1969; Heberle, 1951; Killian & Turner, 1972). An understanding of the movement's current state and future prospects requires that we consider some of its history and leadership and its relationship to the larger society.

SOME ORIGINS OF COMMUNITY MENTAL HEALTH

As noted by both Ozarin and Lemkau, the community mental health movement was the culmination of a series of developments in the mental health field and the society at large.

The passage of the Community Mental Health Centers Act in 1963 was designed to usher in a new era of mental health care and delivery. For many years, there had been gross inequities in the delivery system; adequate care from private practitioners and adequate facilities had been the privilege of the urban and the affluent. Those in the lower classes and residents of the inner city or rural areas either received no care or were shipped off to remote, isolated state mental institutions often depicted as "snake pits" or "human warehouses." To remedy this, the Community Mental Health Centers Act provided for the establishment of a national network of community-based facilities intended to bring adequate care to all. Treatment in these facilities would avoid, if possible, incarceration in antiquated state hospitals.

In addition to community *treatment*, the Community Mental Health Center Act also highlighted the need for the *prevention* of disorder. It was argued that the ubiquity of disorder made even the most ambitious treatment program inadequate to the task. Something had to be done to reduce the incidence of mental illness. This could be accomplished through programs of consultation with community caregivers (e.g., teachers, police, clergy) and through programs of mental health education. A number of leaders in mental health, largely academicians and theoreticians (e.g., Gerald Caplan, Leonard Duhl, Nicholas Hobbs, George Albee, Leopold Bellak, Harris Peck, and William Ryan), saw this legislation as providing the opportunity for the mental health disciplines to exercise an enormous potential for positive social change. CMHCs and CMHC staff would, in addition to treating those already disordered, prevent mental illness in much the same way as public health workers in the previous century had eradicated many infectious diseases.

Poverty, injustice, and racism were seen not only as evils in themselves but also as causes of disorder. Through consultation with community leaders or through the organization and development of the community, salutary change would be brought about. Community mental health was seen as going beyond the traditional one-to-one physican/patient medical model and adopting the population- and prevention-oriented public health model. Hersch (1972) argued that CMHCs could even go beyond the latter and opt for a social action model. Calls were frequently and eloquently sounded for those in the newly created community mental health centers to meet these new challenges and to assume the functions of social activists or agents of social change. These exhortations fit in well with the prevailing reformist and ameliorist *Zeitgeist* of the 1960s.

The decade of the 1960s was one that witnessed the emergence of community mental health as a major focus of the mental health care delivery system. It did not arise de novo. Rather, the community mental health movement was a culmination of a series of developments in the care and treatment of mental disorders that can be traced back to colonial days. These orientations toward the mentally ill were characterized by a series of pendulumlike swings between optimism and pessimism about "curability." Additionally, the ascendancy of the CMHC in the 1960s was closely related to a series of medical and sociopolitical developments at that time. The idea of the "therapeutic community" (Jones, 1976) was based on the notion that the demoralization and estrangement often exhibited by mental patients could be overcome through utilizing the social structure of the hospital (see Gruenberg, Chapter 13, this volume). Advances in psychopharmacology made possible the easier management and early release of many patients (Ochberg & Ozarin, 1976; Pasamanick et al., 1967). Finally, many state hospitals were reorganized in ways that reduced their isolation from the communities from which their patients came (Bloom, 1975). (For a more detailed discussion of the sociopolitical and historical developments, see Bloom, 1975; Bockoven, 1969;

Ewalt & Ewalt, 1969; Felix, 1957; Musto, 1975; Ochberg & Ozarin, 1976; Rossi, 1962; Snow & Newton, 1976; Lemkau, Chapter 1, this volume; and Ozarin, Chapter 2, this volume.)

A helpful concept in understanding community mental health is that of a movement. This term suggests an organized effort, with a discernible leadership and ideology. A particular movement, if it is to be understood in other than purely internal terms, must be seen in its larger sociocultural context.

Levine and Levine (1970) have characterized the relationship between a movement and its milieu. They argue that any given period may be seen as either politically conservative or reformist. In a conservative atmosphere, problems are seen as the result of individual defect, and their solutions are intrapsychic. On the other hand, in a reformist period, problems are seen as due to structural defect, and solutions involve changes in the society. These represent ideal types, and no period is characterized exclusively by any single approach.

Dorothea Dix's efforts to improve the lot of the mentally ill in the 19th century was not an isolated crusade. Rather, it was part of a larger social consciousness that included women's suffrage, prison reform, and the abolition of slavery.

The 1960s counterpart of this earlier "social consciousness" that helped bring community mental health to fruition was ushered in with the election of President Kennedy in 1960. The "New Frontier" envisaged by the Kennedy Administration was predicated in part on the notion that serious social inequities existed and that these could be ameliorated or eliminated through programs of federal legislation and intervention. One of the seminal works in social science that helped raise societal consciousness about poverty was Michael Harrington's *The Other America* (1962). In it, he graphically portrayed the dimensions and consequences of poverty in both urban and rural areas. The major federal response in this area was the "War on Poverty." This was greatly expanded in the Johnson Administration. It was felt that a massive infusion of money could eliminate poverty as a national problem (see Moynihan, 1969).

The impact of the Supreme Court's desegregation decision in 1954 was slow to be felt, but it signaled a change in the pace and direction of the Civil Rights Movement. Federal intervention on behalf of school desegregation began in the Eisenhower Administration and was rapidly broadened and accelerated under Kennedy and Johnson.

In addition to federal efforts, there were voter registration drives. The Peace Corps and VISTA were major efforts to direct idealistic and humanitarian motives of Americans toward improving both this country and the world. Hughes (1969: 63) captured the temper of the times while noting:

> This third post-war generation among the young recalled the first in its concern for public issues: it alternated protests against racial segregation with activities in the cause of peace. Its heroes were the civil rights workers, white and black, who went into the South in successive summers, a few of whom paid for their devotion with their lives. It took courage from the sense that President Kennedy imparted that the nation was once more on the move. Commitment to humanity became its imperative, "We Shall Overcome" its anthem, fraternity and good will its modes of moral expression. It sought to refrain from hatred, and its tactics were invariably nonviolent.

Later on in the decade, both the Civil Rights Movement and liberal social reform efforts became increasingly militant. The Civil Rights Movement shifted toward a broader concern with the disadvantaged status of Orientals, Indians, and Latinos, as well as Blacks. Calls for reform became demands for basic institutional restructuring and, in its most extreme manifestation, revolution.

Hollingshead and Redlich (1958), Leighton (1959), and Srole et al. (1962), demonstrated that mental illness and the social structure were closely related. Mental illness of a more serious variety was more commonly found in the lowest stratum of the society. Exacerbating the situation, the poor were least likely to receive adequate treatment (e.g., Riessman et al., 1964). If mental disorder of a more serious variety was more likely to be found among the poor and the disadvantaged, then it might be that poverty and mental disorder were etiologically associated. Also, racism could be seen as implicated here, since Blacks, Chicanos, and other racial and ethnic minorities were disproportionately found among the poor.

The state hospitals had been founded in the previous century in a spirit of reformist zeal and optimism. For some time, however, they had deteriorated and were in a deplorable state of decay: overcrowded, understaffed, and offering little or no treatment. Journalistic exposés (e.g., Deutsch, 1948) focused on the state to which they had sunk.

As Roland Warren (1971) has noted, in a complex society such as ours, very little by way of purposive social change can be accomplished in the absence of federal intervention. The community mental health movement became actualized through federal legislation initiatives that have been described both here and elsewhere (see Bloom, 1975; Chu & Trotter, 1973; Musto, 1975; Ochberg & Ozarin, 1976). As indicated earlier, the federal government's role in mental health began in earnest in 1946 with the passage of legislation establishing the National Institute of Mental Health (NIMH). NIMH was given the charge of facilitating research and training in mental health and in improving the quality of community-based programs. Subsequent legislation enabled the NIMH to assist mental hospitals directly in the upgrading of their programs and also established the influential Joint Commission on Mental Health and Illness. The Joint Commission conducted extensive surveys on a number of dimensions of the problem of mental disorder, and its report, *Action for Mental Health* (1961), contained a number of recommendations. These called for an expanded federal role in mental health service training and delivery, with the major emphasis being on the provision of services in a community context. At the same time, other groups within the Department of Health, Education and Welfare were charged with the responsibility for planning for new mental health services (see Ozarin, Chapter 2, this volume).

When the report of the Joint Commission reached the desk of President Kennedy, a cabinet-level task force was appointed to prepare a set of legislative recommendations. The President asked the Secretary of DHEW, together with the Secretary of Labor and the Administrator of Veteran's Affairs, to undertake an analysis of the Joint Commission Report and suggest possible courses of action. The President drew heavily on this report for preparation of his 1963 special message on mental health and mental retardation that proposed legislation to Congress in which he urged the creation of a comprehensive community mental health system. These recommendations were embodied in the historic call by President Kennedy for a "bold new approach" to the care and treatment of the mentally ill through the establishment of a new mode of mental health service delivery: the Community Mental Health Center. The legislation envisaged the establishment of a national network of centers, each with a defined area of responsibility, offering mental health services to the entire population. The original goal was the establishment of a national network of 2,000 centers.

As indicated previously, these CMHCs would remedy the inequities in mental health services delivery. By serving all persons in a catchment area, affluence would not be a criterion for treatment. By locating CMHCs in previously underserved inner city and rural areas, geography would no longer be a barrier. Finally, by treating the patient in the community, one could avoid the pernicious effects of lengthy institutionalization in custodial hospitals.

In sum, the passage of the Community Mental Health Centers Act in 1963 and the process of establishing a national network of CMHCs represented the formalization of a complex series of developments within the mental health professions and of certain broader ameliorative currents within the larger society. Their coalescence took a particular form: "The Third Psychiatric Revolution."

THE CONCEPTUAL BASIS OF COMMUNITY MENTAL HEALTH

President John F. Kennedy launched the Community Mental Health Centers Program by sending a message on mental illness and mental retardation to Congress on February 5, 1963. In that message he outlined the severity of the problem and its overwhelming cost, not only in dollars for the care of those affected, but also in human suffering and the loss of human resources.

In his message, Kennedy proposed a "bold new approach" that would substitute comprehensive community care for custodial institutional care. He requested that the Congress enact legislation to "1) authorize grants to the States for construction of comprehensive community mental health centers . . . 2) authorize short-term project grants for initial staffing costs of comprehensive community mental health centers . . . and 3) facilitate the preparation of community plans for these new facilities as a necessary preliminary to any construction or staffing assistance."

The community mental health center movement started as a restructuring of the locus of mental health services and evolved into a major mental health service delivery system for the United States. The key concepts responsible for this restructuring of the mental health delivery system were: geographic responsibility, comprehensiveness, continuity, accessibility, responsiveness, community involvement, and prevention.

Geographic Responsibility. To establish a community-based service, a CMHC became responsible for a well-defined population residing in close proximity to the center. Through its mental health plan, each State Mental Health Authority subdivided its state into geographical areas (catchment areas) of from 75,000 to 200,000 persons. Each catchment area (CA) was, therefore, the center of a community and entitled to have one federally supported community mental health center within its boundaries. This was to avoid fragmentation, ensure accountability, and promote coordination among mental health service providers in the area. Thus, all residents of the CA, regardless of age, sex, race, ethnicity, diagnosis, or ability to pay had to be served by the CMHC. In addition, the concept of geographic responsibility was to assure that CMHCs became systems of care, rather than just a new service provider. To be fully effective, a CMHC had to identify other mental health service providers in the CA and attempt to develop affiliation agreements with them so as to provide the residents with as comprehensive a range of mental health services as possible. Required services not existing in the service area had to be developed by the center. Thus, the concept of geographic responsibility carried with it the implications of comprehensiveness, continuity of care, accessibility, and responsiveness on which the entire CMHC program was founded.

Comprehensiveness. Comprehensiveness in the CMHC program was interpreted as requiring a center to provide whatever mental health services were needed by anyone residing in the CA, regardless of age, sex, race, ethnicity, diagnosis, or ability to pay. The service range was divided on a time continuum and given service designations depending on when and for how long care was to be provided. Thus, consultation and education services were considered part of the services to be provided prior to the need by residents for direct services. It was to assist other service providers in the community to handle potential mental health problems and thus forestall or avoid the need for direct mental health services. It was also to assist the public in its understanding of mental health problems so that it might improve its ability to cope with problems that might, without such understanding, lead to the need for direct mental health services. Twenty-four-hour, seven-day-a-week emergency services were to be available for immediate responsiveness on the part of the center to the need for mental health services of an acute nature. Outpatient services were to provide whatever was needed by residents on an ongoing basis with minimum disruption to continuing occupational, social, and personal activities.

Partial hospitalization required more hours of care and greater frequency than outpatient services and was intended to help residents who needed mental services during periods of the day or week when they were most vulnerable to their mental health problems. Thus, for those who could not cope temporarily with their usual daytime activities but had no trouble being at home evenings, nights, and weekends, there was day care. For those who could cope with regular daytime and possibly occupational activities, but who needed the security of understanding mental health personnel evenings, nights, and weekends, there was the night hospital. For those that could make it during the week but found the weekend and holidays overwhelming, there was the weekend hospital. Inpatient care on a 24-hour basis was provided for those so overwhelmed by their mental health problems that they required a secure mental health setting until they could muster sufficient psychological strength to require a lesser time frame of care. Most persons were expected to achieve this relatively quickly after the acute phase of their distress had passed.

These time sequences of care were each designated as an essential service of the comprehensive program the CMHC was to provide. The essential services, therefore, covered everything that has since been elaborated into additional services by specifying the target groups to be served. The basic philosophy of the community mental health center movement excluded no group from being served. It was expected that the essential services to be provided by a center were for all persons residing in the catchment area, without specifying whether they were children, the elderly, alcoholic and drug abusers, or the chronically mentally ill.

Continuity of Care. In the fragmented, pre-CMHC service arrangement, where a number of independent providers existed in a community, a person could go from one service provider to another without any continuity of care. Each clinic, hospital, or private practitioners would often repeat intake procedures and examinations and have no, or minimal, knowledge of what had been learned previously. The concept of continuity of care stems from the intent that community mental health centers be coordinated networks of services. Therefore, once a person entered the system, there was to be no need for new entrance examinations by other parts of the system should the person be referred there. Records and, if possible, therapists were to follow the person through the system, whether in the crisis center, the outpatient clinic, the day care service, or on an impatient ward.

Accessibility. The community mental health center concept of accessibility was to assure all persons residing in the center's CA the advantage of receiving the mental health services they needed when they needed them. The intent of the limited geographical area served by the center was to make it accessible to persons by being located within a reasonably close proximity to where they lived. Where the geographic area was very large, CMHCs were to develop satellites so that service locations would still be within reasonable distances. Geographic accessibility, however, was only one aspect of this concept. It also covered economic, cultural, psychological, and temporal accessibility. The tenet that services should be available to persons regardless of ability to pay was basic to the philosophy of the community mental health center program. Its implementation has been difficult due to the fiscal problems and reimbursement constraints that CMHCs have experienced. Cultural accessibility's intent was for center services to be relevant to the diverse cultural groups residing in CAs. In like manner, psychological accessibility was concerned with the attitudes, feelings, and nature of the CMHC's setting and the impact of these factors on persons seeking services. Lastly, the services were to be accessible in terms of the times that they were offered. Evening and weekend hours of operation were intended to take care of this aspect of accessibility.

Responsiveness. This concept is closely related to accessibility but was expected to address the nature of the services provided rather than whether or not persons could obtain them. This concept was particularly important for centers that had minority or non-English-speaking populations in their CAs.

Community Involvement. A major strength of the CMHC program has been its emphasis on community involvement. This was intended primarily to assure responsiveness. In addition, it was hoped that it would develop the necessary public support for the center, to enable it to continue operations after the termination of federal support.

Prevention. An important emphasis of the community mental health center movement was concern for the mental health of the community as a whole, not just individual residents. CMHCs were expected to work with other community agencies to help develop mental health-engendering programs for persons residing in the area. This was considered part of the mission of the center's consultation and education services. These concepts have helped to change the mental health services delivery system in the United States and have played an important part in changing the staffing patterns of many mental health service organizations.

THE EVOLUTION OF COMMUNITY MENTAL HEALTH–LEGISLATIVE MILESTONES

The CMHC program was implemented by Congress in its enactment of the Community Mental Health Centers Act

(PL88-164) in 1963. In the next 18 years, the original legislation was amended substantially. This resulted in a considerably expanded and altered program. The most recent legislation—the Omnibus Reconciliation Act of 1981—dramatically redirected and reduced the nature of community-based mental health services. This section will consider the rise and fall of community mental health through these legislative changes.

The legislation that launched the CMHC movement was the Community Mental Health Centers Act of 1963, signed by the President on October 31, 1963. House Reports No. 694 and 862 and Senate Report No. 180 were the basis for this legislation. In the course of the legislative development, grants for the support of professional and technical staff at community mental health centers were deleted and the final conference report provided only for grants for construction. Authorized to be appropriated as grants for the construction and equipment of public and other nonprofit community mental health centers was $35 million for the fiscal year ending June 30, 1965, $50 million for the fiscal year ending June 30, 1966, and $65 million for the fiscal year ending June 30, 1967. For each fiscal year, the allotments were made from the sums appropriated to the states on a percentage basis of population, extent of need, and financial need. The construction of facilities was partially financed by funds authorized by the act. Matching monies were to be provided by state and local sources.

Each state was to designate a single state agency (SSA) as the sole agency for the administration or supervision of the administration of a state plan. Many states designated construction-type agencies—others designated mental health service agencies.

State plans were to be submitted for approval. They were to identify CAs of from 75,000 to 200,000 persons. The plans were to provide a statewide system of "adequate Community Mental Health Centers," and with consideration of relationships to other planning programs, priority was given to general hospitals that wished to develop a CMHC as part of their services.[1] Each center was required to provide for a minimum of services including inpatient, outpatient, partial hospitalization, emergency, consultation, and education. Facilities were to be individually designed for the needs of the CA. Funds were to be used for the construction of new buildings, expansion of existing facilities, completion of shell space, initial fixed equipment, and movable equipment and furnishings, including transportation vehicles and architectural fees. One or more buildings could be built; the various services of a center program did not have to be under one roof.

In 1968, 1970, and 1974, the original legislation was amended to allow increasing reimbursement for construction costs. Almost all the awards made under the provisions of the act have resulted in either the construction of or otherwise obtaining a facility for use by a CMHC to provide mental health services in its CA. Many grants encompassed buildings located in separate facilities throughout a CA. Each facility has been designed for the characteristics of the clients, staff, and programs, as well as for the customs and climate of the CA. Each CMHC facility has been designed and constructed to meet specific CA needs. Thus, they are each different and, through their design, responsive to their communities.

In 1965, Congress amended the original Act (PL89-105). The intent of this amendment was to expand the system in a number of ways. First, funds were made available on a declining basis for professional and technical staff. In addition, PL89-105 clarified some issues that had arisen regarding eligibility for staffing grants, consonance of the CMHCs' services with comprehensive state mental health plans, and requirements for services.

The tempo of CMHC expansion accelerated rapidly. As of June 30, 1968, the NIMH had awarded staffing grants to 331 new CMHCs in a diverse cross-section of communities nationwide. Of these new centers, 76 had received both a staffing and a construction grant, 175 of the remainder had received only a construction grant, and 80 had received only a staffing grant. Of the staffing grants, 12 percent had been awarded to centers with previous staffing grants, assisting these centers in expanding their mental health service programs. Additionally, centers had the opportunity to adjust staffing patterns through supplemental grants enabling them to expand personnel as unforeseen needs arose, while raising salaries to competitive levels when necessary for recruitment purposes. The bulk of applicants (75 percent) for initial and supplemental staffing grants were general hospitals. Special purpose corporations, set up to deliver mental health services, independent mental health clinics, and public mental hospitals accounted for the remaining applicants. By 1981, with 763 operational centers, about one-half of the country had geographic accessibility to a CMHC.

The availability of staffing grants for the initial costs of professional and technical personnel significantly influenced the responsiveness and availability of community mental health services to communities nationwide. Services were made accessible to large numbers of persons and communities previously excluded from care. Various program reviews indicated that the relationships between CMHCs and public hospitals had undergone considerable modification, as well as changes in the number and types of patients being treated in these facilities. Continuity of care was being facilitated by sufficient staffing patterns at CMHCs that permitted the establishment and operation of effective and efficient community aftercare programs. CMHCs were monitored annually by the federal government. Continuity of care was an important element of the CMHC program and therefore was reviewed carefully. Site visitors examined records, talked to staff and patients, and read center policies. While lacking empirical data on continuity of care, the reviewers found that continuity of care was viewed as a primary element in the delivery of quality CMHC services.

These amendments provided additional momentum in establishing community-based mental health services. The range and depth of services in CMHCs have expanded considerably, while the resident populations of state and local public mental hospitals have declined. In 1955 there were 559,000 residents of state and county mental hospitals, but by 1974 only 146,000 were residents (USDHHS, 1981b).

The CMHC Amendments of 1970 (PL91-211) were enacted on March 13, 1970. This legislation further extended the scope of center services. It provided funds for the initiation and development of services to rural and poverty areas, extended the duration of staffing grants, and provided incentives for the development of consultation and children's services.

There were a number of new program directions authorized in these amendments to meet urgent needs that were identified during the rapid growth and development of the centers' program. For the first time, recognition was given to the need for a longer start-up period and to the special needs of urban and rural poverty areas. Both concepts, strengthened by later amendments, have been highly important to establishing CMHCs in previously unserved and underserved areas.

Another "first" was the focus on the needs of children in a separate grant program. This proved to be a highly successful and useful grant mechanism designed to reach out to children in their normal family and neighborhood life setting and to provide innovative approaches for both the coordination and integration of existing human services resources for children in the community and for the collaborative organization and delivery of services by CMHCs with other community child and family health services.

Of importance too was the new Initiation and Development Grant mechanism for urban or rural poverty areas. This program enabled communities without the necessary resources to assess their local needs for mental health services, to design appropriate programs to meet those needs, and to develop the necessary community, professional, and fiscal support necessary to implement such a program. These I & D projects served both as "pioneers" and "guinea pigs" for the planning grants that were authorized in the 1975 amendments.

Requiring review of CMHC grant applications by the National Advisory Mental Health Council was also a significant move. Up to this point, the CMHC Grant Review Committee, made up of central office staff members of various divisions of the National Institute of Mental Health, carried out the task of review. The requirement for council review came at a time when President Nixon had begun to chip away at the CMHC program. Review by a group of national experts proved to be a unifying element in the development and maintenance of national standards for the CMHC program, thereby helping to counter the Nixon forces aimed at its elimination.

At the time the 1970 CMHC Amendments were being enacted, major administrative aspects of the CMHC grant programs were decentralized to the ten DHEW regional offices. In effect, this created a central office role of planning and program development (with the National Advisory Mental Health

Council responsible for quality control) and delegated to the field the day-to-day operations. The spirit of this reorganization reflected a national mood of "bringing the government closer to the people." Sufficient resources for carrying out this complex program and difficulties in coordinating the ten regional operations were the negative aspects of this approach. On the positive side were the closer interactions of the regional office staff with state and local groups.

President Nixon viewed the CMHC program as a demonstration program. As such, he felt that it had demonstrated its utility and that states should pick up the responsibility for service provision. This was part and parcel of Nixon's views on block grants and state's roles. While Nixon did not initiate a block grant program, he did begin a revenue-sharing program as a first step in that direction. (States, however, were unsure about the continuity of this money and hence put these monies primarily into capital investment rather than into programs that would have ongoing financial commitments.)

Congress and the White House differed when it came to the CMHC program. While Nixon saw this as a program that should be abolished and picked up by states, Congress took the position that this was an excellent program that they wished to continue to fund. The preamble to the 1975 Amendments (PL94-63) clearly stated Congress' intent:

TITLE III–COMMUNITY MENTAL HEALTH CENTERS

(a) The Congress finds that–

(1) community mental health care is the most effective and humane form of care for a majority of mentally ill individuals;

(2) the federally funded community mental health centers have had a major impact on the improvement of mental health care by–

(A) fostering coordination and cooperation between various agencies responsible for mental health care which in turn has resulted in a decrease in overlapping services and more efficient utilization of available resources,

(B) bringing comprehensive community mental health care to all in need within a specific geographic area regardless of ability to pay, and

(C) developing a system of care which insures continuity of care for all patients,

and thus are a national resource to which all Americans should enjoy access; and

(3) there is currently a shortage and maldistribution of quality community health care resources in the United States.

(b) The Congress further declares that Federal funds should continue to be made available for the purposes of initiating new and continuing existing community mental health centers and initiating new services within existing centers, and for the monitoring of the performance of all federally funded centers to insure their responsiveness to community needs and national goals relating to community mental health care.

Congress mandated in PL94-63 what had previously been requirements in regulations and policy. It was felt that there was a need to be specific with regard to special population groups in the law. Congress appropriated additional funds. However, these sums were never authorized.

Though President Nixon resigned, President Ford followed through on the Nixon White House policy and vetoed PL94-63. Congress overrode the veto, and the bill was passed (Spaner, 1982).

It should be noted here that the Reagan Administration's views on block grants and state responsibility can be traced back to the Nixon Administration.

Probably the most significant provision of PL94-63 was a major expansion of the scope of community mental health. In addition to the original five, CMHCs were now required to supply a total of 12 services, including services for children and the elderly, screening services, followup care, transitional services, and services for alcohol and drug abusers.

In addition, new grant mechanisms were provided for the support of planning, initial operations, consultation/education, conversion, financial distress, and facilities. These grants replaced staffing, construction, and the specialty grants for alcohol treatment, drug abuse, and services for children.

Studies such as the one conducted by the General Accounting Office (GAO, 1974) indicated that many CMHCs were deficient in the area of program management. Accordingly, in Sec 206(e) of the 1975 amendments, Congress authorized the Two Percent Technical Assistance Program. Under this program 2 percent of the appropriations for any fiscal year were to be set aside to provide technical assistance for program management and for training in program management of CMHCs receiving grants.

PL94-63, by supporting a portion of the cost of initial operations, provided opportunities for the establishment of new centers in areas that were in need of mental health services but which otherwise would not have been able to initiate such services. A second effect was increased participation by citizens and their representatives in the development, operation, and evaluation of CMHC programs, thus making them more responsive to local needs. A third effect occurred in the capability of CMHCs to evaluate their programs and institute procedures for quality assurance and peer review. There has also been marked improvement in the ability of CMHCs to use administrative management knowledge provided through the Two Percent Technical Assistance Program.

An additional area in which there has been changes is in the relationship of CMHCs to other health service providers. One example of this development is a joint program between the NIMH and the Bureau of Community Health Services, where they are funding CMHC staff persons to work full-time at several community health centers providing consultation to the primary health care providers, assist in mental health triage, and to provide client services.[2]

As we have indicated, the major amendments to the Community Mental Health Centers Act after its initial enactment in 1963 occurred in 1965, 1970, and 1975. However, throughout the history of the legislation there have been extensions and changes reflecting the evolution and expansion of the CMHC service delivery system. Essentially, the CMHC legislation was amended on an almost yearly basis from 1963 to 1979. These changes expanded the scope of CMHC services, particularly in the area of alcohol and drugs and extended appropriations for construction and staffing. These amendments also called for changes in center governance and modified certain fiscal requirements.

The amendments enlarging the fiscal base and scope of CMHCs indicated a base of congressional support. The executive branch, however, was less supportive. As we noted earlier, both Presidents Nixon and Ford attempted to modify CMHC services substantially.

While still Governor of Georgia, Jimmy Carter was supportive of the mental health efforts and particularly of the CMHC program. It is not surprising that one of his first acts on becoming president was to sign an executive order (No. 11973) on February 17, 1977, establishing the President's Commission on Mental Health (PCMH), with Rosalyn Carter as honorary chairperson. In 1978, the PCMH published its report (PCMH, 1978). While reaffirming a commitment to the principle of community-based mental health services, the report broke some new ground.

The period in which President Carter initiated his commission was also the time that advocates for the chronically mentally ill were beginning to voice their opinion regarding the failures of CMHCs in meeting their needs. Also, the commission came along at a time when many states were sending along messages regarding the fact that CMHC staffing grants went directly to local areas and were bypassing state government. Many states felt that they ought to be involved in mental health planning. The swing of the pendulum that began in the Nixon period toward more state control of social programs was increasingly moving in the direction away from federal control and toward more state involvement.

The Mental Health Systems Act reflects this swing. While it still mandated federal grants, it also initiated a partnership with states.

Spaner (1982) views this swing toward block grants as a sort of reaction formation against the Johnson Administration's policies. The swing of the political pendulum, however, took some time to develop momentum. The Mental Health Systems Act was the culmination of these changes.

The Mental Health Systems Act (PL96-398) was signed by President Carter on October 7, 1980. It was the first major change in mental health legislation in 17 years, and it is an ironic note that it was never implemented.

The Systems Act renewed a federal commitment to the establishment of a network of community-based mental health services in the context of special emphases on services for the most vulnerable and dependent groups of mentally ill persons, especially those who are chronically mentally ill, children, and the elderly. The act also called for attention to the needs of rural and minority populations, and for closer links between health and mental health services. At the same time, the act broke new ground by defining a performance-based partnership among federal, state, and local agencies.

The long-range national goal for mental health services embodied in the 1963 CMHC legislation was based on the principle that comprehensive, community-based care should be accessible to all persons in need. The Systems Act was designed to continue progress toward this goal. Its themes included community-based mental health services that were comprehensive, flexible, accountably organized and funded, and coordinated with health and related social support and welfare services. Mental health services are the heart of a system of high quality care that is accessible to all and uniquely responsive to each. The major features of the Systems Act were: continued support of the CMHC program; authorization of grants for programs providing both mental health and related support services for three highly vulnerable groups of mentally ill persons (the chronically mentally ill, severely distrubed children and adolescents, and elderly persons); and flexible new opportunities for the most needy areas to receive federal support for programs providing a core set of community-based services for these same high-risk groups or for other populations with unmet needs—for example, the urban and rural poor, and ethnic and racial minorities.

Other major themes of this legislation related to its restructuring of federal/state/local participation in the building of coordinated mental health services systems in states and communities. A framework was established for an innovative process of cooperation and shared responsibility that focused on developing states' capabilities. States were accorded considerable leverage to design and administer programs for building statewide systems of mental health care.

The act also strengthened requirements related to planning and accountability. This theme spoke to the concern for maximum effective use of scarce resources and the need for a more coherent and cohesive organization of services. Included here were provisions mandating the negotiation of a "performance contract," with every program as a condition of federal funding. Standards and schedules were to be specified, and the roles and responsibilities of each party to the contract were to be spelled out.

Ronald Reagan was elected president on a platform that called for a substantially reduced role of the federal government. Consequently, many health and human services programs were affected, some being either eliminated entirely or having funds cut back drastically; others were turned over to the states with some federal funds being given via block grants. The Mental Health Systems Act was one of the pieces of legislation that was rescinded.

On August 13, 1981, President Reagan signed into law PL97-35, The Omnibus Reconciliation Act in which the Mental Health Systems Act was repealed. Where previously there had been 25 separate HHS-run spending programs, each with its set of federal regulations, this legislation streamlined those 25 programs into seven block grants to states. The purpose of block grants is to achieve greater flexibility in the use of funds, thereby improving the efficient use of tax dollars and cost effectiveness of services to recipients. The blocks are: preventive health; maternal and child health; alcohol, drug abuse, and mental health; primary care; social services; community services; and energy assistance.

The Alcohol, Drug Abuse, and Mental Health Block Grant (ADM) provides funds to states to establish and maintain programs to combat alcohol and drug abuse, to care for the mentally ill, and to promote mental health. The major purposes of this block grant are: the support of programs to control and prevent alcoholism and drug abuse; the support of community treatment services for mental and emotional illness through community mental health centers; provisions for the rehabilitation of alcohol and drug abusers and the mentally ill; and a services emphasis on outpatient care for the chronically mentally ill.

The block grants consolidated several federal grant programs. These include: mental health services; drug abuse project grants; drug abuse state formula grants; alcoholism project grants; and alcoholism state formula grants.

Since this legislation is new, it would be useful to note some of its special provisions. The block grant limits administrative costs to a maximum of 10 percent.

Unlike previous legislation, reporting requirements are not extensive. In a required annual application, each state must certify compliance with 13 assurances of quality, fairness, and appropriateness of expenditure. State legislature hearings are required, beginning with the second year of block operation. The states are also required to prepare proposed spending plans and to make them available for public comment. In addition, postexpenditure reports, available for public inspection, are also required.

The block grant contains maintenance of effort provisions requiring states to make grants to all community mental health centers that received grants in FY80, unless the Secretary of HHS agrees to defunding. Initially, funds are to be divided between the three ADM components in the same fashion as in FY80. In FY83, 95 percent must be so allocated, and by FY84, 85 percent.

For alcohol and drug abuse projects, at least 35 percent must go to alcohol abuse programs; at least 35 percent to drug abuse programs; and at least 20 percent of the total must be spent on prevention programs.

Although no formal state matching is required, federal funds must supplement spending by state or local government and cannot supplant such spending.

The time for transition from federal to state control was relatively short. States were authorized to take over control of the block grant as early as October 1, 1981. In order to receive federal funds beyond FY82, however, they must assume responsibility no later than October 1, 1982.

In this section, we have traced the evolution of the community mental health legislation. We have also noted that the scope of community mental health became increasingly broad over the years, from five to twelve essential services. The Mental Health Systems Act represented a redirection of the delivery system. The Omnibus Reconciliation Act of 1981, as part of the Reagan Administration's philosophy of a new federalism, has completely reversed the direction of the past 20 years. The implications of this will be considered in the last section. Before looking at the future of community mental health services, however, we have to consider the way in which they have developed. This will be the concern of the next section.

THE EVOLUTION OF COMMUNITY MENTAL HEALTH—CENTER GROWTH AND PATIENT ADDITIONS

The previous sections of this chapter have dealt with some of the sociohistorical background of community health and its evolution as seen through legislative development. Here, we will consider the evolution of community mental health in terms of the growth of the CMHCs and changes in patterns of service, delivery, and patient care. The basic questions to be considered are: Has community mental health made an impact on the mental health care delivery system? and Have the aims of the architects of community mental health been realized?

To begin with, it is evident that a fundamental, if not *the* fundamental goal of community mental health, was to correct the serious imbalance in the mental health care delivery system and to provide care for those who had previously been unserved or underserved. In addition, as we have noted earlier, the state hospitals were in a deplorable state and it was anticipated that inpatient care would be more commonly employed in the patient's community. Some sense of the change wrought by the "Third Psychiatric Revolution" can be seen in the following:

> In 1955, three-quarters of the 1.7 million episodes of care delivered in mental health facilities were inpatient care. . . . Twenty years later, community-based (outpatient and partial care) had replaced hospitalization as the modality of care for almost three-quarters of the 6.9 million episodes of care provided in the United States [USDHEW, 1978: 7].

In other words, in two decades the number of patient care episodes had quadrupled and the locus of care had been almost totally reversed. Put another way, by 1977, CMHCs accounted for nearly one-third of all patient care episodes–both inpatient and outpatient (Witkin, 1980).

More detail on the growth of CMHCs can be seen in Table 3.1.[3]

In 1968, slightly over one-quarter of a million patients were under care in 165 operating CMHCs. Ten years later, there were 600 operating CMHCs caring for 2,136,711 persons–an increase greater than sixfold. The increase in patients under care was not a simple function of the increase in the number of centers, since during this period the average number of patients per CMHC more than doubled.

As one might expect, the rate of increase was not uniform. The early years of CMHC expansion produced greater proportional increases in both patient additions and total number of patients under care. In the years for which data are available, patient additions increased 554 percent, while patients under care showed an almost sevenfold increase (686 percent).

Two of the goals of community mental health were to provide service in the patient's community and to minimize hospitalization in state hospitals. Data in Table 3.2 provide some evidence to support this. The greatest increases in service modality were in partial care days (525 percent–from

Table 3.1
Number of Persons Added and Persons Under Care (Unduplicated) in Federally Funded Community Mental Health Centers, United States, 1968-1978

		Additions during Year		*Patients under Care*	
Year	*Number of Operating CMHCs*	*Total*	*Average per CMHC*	*Total*	*Average per CMHC*
1968	165	180,510	1,094	271,590	1,646
1969	205	254,855	1,243	373,097	1,820
1970	255	334,760	1,313	517,661	2,030
1971	295	432,640	1,467	693,260	2,350
1972	325	511,706	1,574	846,336	2,604
1973	400	652,652	1,632	1,094,430	2,736
1974	434	771,821	1,778	1,322,832	3,048
1975	528	919,037	1,741	1,618,746	3,066
1976	548	1,016,113	1,854	1,877,676	3,426
1977	563	1,048,211	1,862	1,881,798	3,342
1978	600	1,180,800	1,968	2,136,711	3,561

SOURCE: Budget Cards, Office of Liaison and Program Analysis, Mental Health Services Division, NIMH, 1980.

1,151,950 in 1970 to 7,206,301 in 1978—and in outpatient visits—from under 3 million in 1970 to almost 10 million in 1978—an increase of 242 percent. During this same period, inpatient hospitalization increased only 111 percent. These apparent increases actually mask an important trend. When we take into account concomitant growth in the number of CMHCs and consider average per-CMHC, inpatient days actually declined 10 percent (from 7544 to 6772), while partial care and outpatient services increased 165 percent and 45 percent, respectively. It seems reasonable, then, to conclude that inpatient care has been reduced and that more community-based modalities have been increased.

Tables 3.1 and 3.2 illustrate the growth of CMHCs. Also to be noted is the parallel decline of the state hospital as a source of care. In 1955, 49 percent of the 1.7 million patient care episodes were delivered at state and county mental hospitals. By

Table 3.2
Number of Units of Service Provided, by Modality, Federally Funded Community Mental Health Centers, United States, 1970-1978

Year	*Number of Operating CMHCs*	*Inpatient Days*	*Partial Care Days*	*Outpatient Visits (Indiv., Family, Group)*
		Annual Number of Units of Service		
1970	255	1,923,720	1,151,950	2,839,644
1971	295	2,225,396	1,283,330	3,375,705
1972	325	2,561,633	1,928,283	3,902,716
1973	400	3,275,630	2,630,002	5,202,016
1974	434	3,836,452	3,420,981	6,055,759
1975	528	3,948,466	4,237,660	7,596,434
1976	548	3,951,001	5,070,300	8,669,115
1977	563	3,818,497	6,240,461	8,934,220
1978	600	4,063,176	7,206,301	9,724,305
		Average Per CMHC		
1970	255	7544.0	4517.5	11,135.9
1971	295	7543.7	4350.3	11,443.1
1972	325	7881.9	5933.2	12,008.4
1973	400	8189.1	6575.0	13,005.0
1974	434	8839.8	7859.4	13,953.4
1975	528	7478.2	8025.9	14,387.2
1976	548	7209.9	9252.4	15,819.6
1977	563	6782.4	11,084.3	15,869.0
1978	600	6772.0	12,010.5	16,207.2

SOURCE: Inventory of Comprehensive Community Mental Health Centers, Survey and Reports Branch, Division of Biometry and Epidemiology, NIMH unpublished data, 1980.

1975, this figure had dropped to 9 percent of 6.4 million episodes (USDHEW, 1978). In absolute terms, in 1955, 833,000 episodes of care were in these hospitals; by 1975, these had declined to 576,000. CMHCs had emerged and accounted for 2 million episodes of care, as well as having had a major influence on the way services were delivered. This suggests that the locus of care had shifted from the hospital to the community, and that the CMHC increases were not simply a result of uncovering new patient populations. In addition to services provided by CMHCs, there has been an increase in outpatient service provided by non-CMHCs. By 1975, almost half (47 percent) of the episodes of care were delivered by outpatient psychiatric services (USDHEW, 1978).

CMHCs have not been successful in making services available to all age groups. Age-specific addition rates to CMHCs indicate that the 65+ category has the lowest age-specific addition rates/100,000 CA population: 476.8 for males and 472.2 for females. This is also reflected in indirect services: more than one-third of staff hours were devoted to consultation and education schools or agencies dealing with children, while only 5 percent were allocated to facilities for the elderly. Among the young (under 15), the rate of male additions exceeds that for females, while for the other ages, females exceed males.

The architects of the CMHC movement envisaged a national network of 2,000 centers by 1980. Clearly, this has not been realized. As of September 1981, there were 768 centers that had ever been funded. They represented only about one-half of the established areas in the country. As one might expect, the development of community mental health nationally has been uneven; programs in some states have been more fully implemented than in others.

States and territories varied widely in catchmenting: from 18 percent to 100 percent. No clear pattern seems evident except that the more populous states have been less successful in establishing CMHCs than the less populous, rural areas (see Table 3.3).

The rapid growth and expansion of CMHCs created an urgent demand for additional professional and paraprofessional staff. The chapters by Penn and by Rieman elsewhere in this volume discuss this in some detail. It is sufficient at this point to note that the number of staff at CMHCs increased over 250 percent from 1970 to 1978: from 21,544 to 78,095 (Table 3.4). The various disciplines comprising the staff grew at different rates. Psychology and social work expanded most rapidly: 459 and 325 percent, respectively. The growth of psychiatry and nursing was considerably more modest: 103 and 184 percent, respectively. Indeed, a closer look at the data in Table 3.4 indicates that the average full-time equivalent for psychiatrists has declined 65 percent, and for nurses 10 percent. In contrast, for psychologists and social workers, the increases have been 106 and 45 percent, respectively. The decline in psychiatric manpower in CMHCs—their "flight"—has been viewed with some concern by a number of authors (e.g., Talbot, 1979) as evidence of a "demedicalization" and loss of original purpose and intent. The implications of these trends will be considered in the final section.

No discussion of the development of CMHCs would be complete without some reference to the cost of the program. Since the first grant was made in 1965, $268,552,274 (as of September 30, 1981) has been expended by the federal government on the CMHC program (USDHHS, 1981a). This federal expenditure, however, represents only a small part of money spent on CMHCs. As we indicated in the previous section, federal outlays were intended to be seed money and were made on a declining share basis. From 1969 to 1976, the federal share of CMHC funding has declined from 35 to 27 percent (USDHHS, 1980). As centers have matured, receipts from patient fees and third-party payers during this same period of time have increased from 16 to 30 percent.

Another way of illustrating this seed money concept is to note that for newer CMHCs (in operation less than three years), every federal staffing grant dollar was matched by $1.38 in other monies (state and local government, patient fees, insurance payments, and so forth). In contrast, the more established centers (8+ years) generate $2.65 in revenues from different sources for every federal dollar (USDHHS, 1980). It would appear, then, that the seed money did bear fruit.

COMMUNITY MENTAL HEALTH—A CRITICAL APPRAISAL

Up to this point, we have traced the sociocultural evolution of community mental health, its expansion through successive changes in the 1963 legislation, the increase in the number of

Table 3.3
Distribution of Funded CMHCs by State: 1981

	Total CMHs Funded	*Total Number of CAs*	*Percentage of CAs Funded*		*Total CMHCs Funded*	*Total Number of CAs*	*Percentage of CAs Funded*
TOTALS	*768*	*1,565*					
Alabama	21	25	84%	Nebraska	7	12	58%
Alaska	3	16	19%	Nevada	2	4	50%
Arizona	8	15	53%	New Hampshire	7	10	70%
Arkansas	14	14	100%	New Jersey	24	51	47%
California	53	151	35%	New Mexico	6	8	75%
Colorado	18	21	85%	New York	27	127	21%
Connecticut	8	21	38%	North Carolina	28	41	68%
Delaware	2	4	50%	North Dakota	5	8	62%
District of Columbia	3	4	75%	Ohio	31	79	39%
Florida	37	46	80%	Oklahoma	9	15	60%
Georgia	25	34	74%	Oregon	4	18	22%

Hawaii	6	8	75%	Pennsylvania	45	87	52%
Idaho	7	7	100%	Rhode Island	6	8	75%
Illinois	21	81	26%	South Carolina	15	16	94%
Indiana	24	31	77%	South Dakota	5	7	71%
Iowa	6	23	26%	Tennessee	21	30	70%
Kansas	11	16	69%	Texas	33	81	41%
Kentucky	22	22	100%	Utah	9	11	82%
Louisiana	16	31	52%	Vermont	6	6	100%
Maine	8	8	100%	Virginia	14	38	37%
Maryland	10	30	33%	Washington	11	26	42%
Massachusetts	25	40	62%	West Virginia	10	14	71%
Michigan	23	60	38%	Wisconsin	12	37	32%
Minnesota	7	37	18%	Wyoming	4	7	57%
Mississippi	15	16	94%	Guam	1	1	100%
Missouri	16	36	44%	Puerto Rico	11	20	55%
Montana	5	5	100%	Virgin Islands	1	1	100%

SOURCE: Budget Cards, Office of Liaison and Program Analysis, Mental Health Services Division, NIMH, 1981.

Table 3.4
Staffing Patterns in Federally Funded Community Mental Health Centers, United States, 1970-1979

	Discipline								
Year and Selected Status	*Total all Staff*[a]	*Psychiatrists*	*Physicians (nonpsychiatric)*	*Psychologists (BA & above)*	*Social Workers (BA & above)*	*Reg. Nurses*	*Other Prof.*	*LPNs; Ment. Health Workers*	*Admin, Clerical, Fiscal, Maint. personnel*
Total Staff									
1970	21,544	1,981	325	1,314	2,361	2,344	2,502	6,416	4,301
1971	27,551	2,257	461	1,593	2,834	3,064	4,747	7,101	5,494
1972	33,749	2,524	527	2,331	3,712	3,415	3,541	10,498	7,201
1973[b]	35,490	2,441	473	2,654	4,147	3,532	4,161	10,342	7,740
1974	45,205	2,872	622	3,781	5,251	4,148	5,860	12,325	10,346
1975	52,655	2,968	714	4,685	6,262	4,764	7,225	13,538	12,509
1976	62,479	3,738	652	5,770	7,957	5,761	8,290	14,776	15,535
1977	66,440	3,868	661	6,332	8,512	6,117	9,278	14,891	16,781
1978	70,496	3,908	509	5,875	8,751	6,524	10,345	14,931	19,653
1979	78,095	4,029	732	7,356	10,029	6,658	11,434	16,970	20,887

Average Full-Time Equivalent per CMHC									
1970	c	6.8	0.5	4.9	9.7	9.7	8.9	23.5	c
1971	82.9	5.7	0.8	4.8	9.3	9.9	11.1	22.0	19.3
1972	83.6	5.4	0.8	6.1	10.3	9.2	8.8	23.2	19.8
1973[b]	84.1	4.9	0.6	6.5	10.7	8.5	9.9	22.5	20.2
1974	88.3	4.6	0.7	7.5	11.0	8.7	11.4	22.4	22.0
1975	94.3	4.3	0.7	8.5	12.2	8.9	13.4	22.0	24.2
1976	91.8	4.3	0.5	8.6	12.8	8.7	12.6	20.0	24.3
1977	95.7	4.3	0.5	9.2	13.0	8.9	13.4	20.0	26.4
1978	100.5	4.0	0.3	8.5	13.0	9.7	14.7	20.8	29.3
1979	103.8	4.1	0.6	10.1	14.1	8.8	15.8	20.5	29.8

a. Where figures do not add to the total, discrepancies are due to rounding.

b. In 1973, for the first time, the centers were instructed to report as CMHC staff only those supported by the center's budget, with the exception of trainees and volunteers. This differed from previous years. Interpretations of data for staffing should not fail to consider this factor.

c. Not available.

SOURCE: Inventory of Comprehensive Community Mental Health Centers, Survey and Reports Branch, Division of Biometry and Epidemiology, NIMH unpublished data, 1980.

CMHCs, the number of patients served, and in the pool of mental health manpower. We have shown that the community mental health movement was an outgrowth of earlier developments in mental health that found fertile ground in the ameliorative temper of the 1960s. Its promise as a "bold new approach" helped it to obtain increasing financial support from Congress, as well as marked expansion of scope and responsibility. The data that we have presented indicate that at a minimum, the movement has succeeded inasmuch as there has been a substantial increase in the numbers of persons receiving mental health services.

Still to be considered, however, are some of the failures and shortcomings of community mental health. Along with this and given the realities of the 1980s, what is likely to be the future of community-based mental health services?

By now, use of the phrase "bold new approach" to describe community mental health has achieved a rather hoary status. It does, though, along with "Third Psychiatric Revolution" and "Delivery System of the 1960s," capture some of the optimism, enthusiasm, and promise of the vision of community mental health in earlier years. These phrases, too, contain the germ of some of its major shortcomings. In evaluating the success of any enterprise, it is useful to have some clear indication of what was supposed to be accomplished. In the case of community mental health, this is lacking. Was community mental health to be the vehicle for delivering mental health services to previously unserved or underserved populations? Was it supposed to reduce the pernicious effects of incarceration in distant state hospitals by treating the patient closer to home? Was it, using the public health model, to attempt to prevent mental disorder by altering the sociocultural environment in much the same way that the environmental sanitarians of the 19th century had conquered many infectious diseases? Unfortunately for community mental health, the answer to all of these questions was "yes."

In the first flush of enthusiasm, community mental health's potential was vastly oversold. It would remedy the inequities inherent in the old system, and it would also prevent mental disorder by eliminating those features of the social milieu that were felt to be psychotoxic: poverty, racism, discrimination, war, and so on. By moving from the treatment room and regarding the entire community as patient, community mental health practitioners would alter society in a positive manner. Community mental health would be a panacea for all of society's ills. This is not the appropriate context for an extended discussion of the topic, but it should be noted that these new directions for community mental health did not go unchallenged. Both Burrows (1969) and Dunham (1967) referred to the concept as a "psychiatric bandwagon," while Kolb (1970) chastised his colleagues for their "flight from the patient" and Panzetta (1971) felicitiously referred to it as "psychiatric chutzpah." Extended discussions can be found in Arnhoff (1975), Feldman (1978), Musto (1975), Snow and Newton (1976), Wagenfeld (1972), and Wagenfeld and Robin (1980). The definitive word is yet to be written, but there seems to be no evidence that large-scale efforts by community mental health practitioners to alter the social structure in the name of mental health have been effective (see Lemkau, Chapter 9, this volume).

Community mental health's scope and capabilities were oversold in other ways, too. Dinitz and Beran (1971) have characterized community mental health's tendency to see more and more areas of life as relevant as "boundary-busting." An example of this can be seen in its legislative development. The 1963 legislation mandated five essential services. Over the years, as we have noted, this was broadened considerably until, in the 1975 amendments, 12 services were delineated. With a view of CMHC as a panacea, additional requirements and services were added by the federal government during the Johnson Administration without any thought to feasibility or priority. Congress was supportive of the CMHC program (although authorizations were never as high as appropriations). How CMHCs would actually live up to these "superprogram" goals was not the concern.

Up until PL94-63, Congress believed that the CMHC program was doing good as a result of the observational information given it. PL94-63 was the first effort to obtain more than just observational evaluations (see 1% evaluation clause in PL94-63).

Federal staff did not view themselves as evaluators but rather saw themselves as program developers and consultants. There was always a lot of resistance among regional office staff to monitoring/evaluation, as they viewed this as policing, not consulting. Even when Congress began to see the need for harder data on the CMHC program, the CMHC people did not respond with clear goal setting, priorities, and evaluation studies that showed measurable attainments.

It seems fair and reasonable to suggest that the community mental health program bit off goals much too large to digest. The 1975 amendments went beyond the boundaries of an achievable program. In a surprisingly frank assessment, an NIMH publication noted:

> Through PL94-63, passed in July, 1975, Congress provided for the survival of this "Great Society" program. However, in its enthusiasms for this species of social and medical programming the Congress may have created a modern day dinosaur, i.e., a huge and complex organism which requires nutrients that from a Darwinian perspective far exceed the capacity of the environment to provide [USDHEW, 1978: 64].

In pursuing the chimera of activism and community change, CMHCs often neglected the chronic patients, those most in need of services. Unfortunately, the community mental health program has been deemed a failure by both sides. Liberals and community activists such as the Nader group (Chu & Trotter, 1973) have argued that it has failed because it did not become the human services program that would solve all of society's problems. Others, for example, Zusman and Lamb (1977) see much of the community-based activism as a wasteful squandering of scarce resources. In a situation in which there were never any clearly articulated goals and priorities, it seemed inevitable that this state of affairs would obtain. The report of the President's Commission on Mental Health (1978) and the ensuing Mental Health Systems Act appeared to be a constructive change of direction. While continuing to endorse strongly the principle of community-based services, it specified target groups in particular need of services and indicated that the number of services offered by a center would be determined by community need and not some arbitrary figure. As we have already pointed out, we will never know what might have happened had such recommendations been followed.

Much of the current attack on community mental health is based on political philosophy rather than empirical data. The failure of mental health researchers and evaluators in the 1960s and 1970s to demonstrate clearly the efficacy of community interventions may have contributed to this state of affairs. Community- as opposed to institutionally based care was unquestioningly accepted as superior. While one could not quarrel with the humaneness of this position, the efficacy of this care from an economic point of view was not demonstrated. Cost effectiveness, worker productivity, and related issues were not targeted as important issues for study.

Finally, we have pointed out that the federal dollars invested in community mental health did have a multiplier effect. Still, one would have to point out that many CMHCs continued to view federal funding as a continuing sources of dollars, not taking the eight years of funding/seed money concept seriously. Steps to become financially independent of public and, especially, federal support were not addressed early in the CMHC program.[4]

In sum, it is clear that a series of developments within the mental health community and coming to fruition in the heady optimism and liberalism of the 1960s helped to create a view of community mental health as a panacea. That this did not prove to be the case is clear. The proliferation of required services in the absence of clear federal priorities only added to the problem. Granted that community mental health did not eliminate war, poverty, racism, and injustice in our society, as some of its proponents had hoped. The most critical evaluation, however, cannot lose sight of the fact that one of the major goals of the 1963 legislation—providing mental health services on a catchment area basis to communities and populations previously unserved or underserved—has been realized.

FROM A CLOUDY CRYSTAL BALL–THE FUTURE OF COMMUNITY-BASED MENTAL HEALTH SERVICES

The implementation of the Omnibus Reconciliation Act (PL97-35) on October 1, 1981 represented a complete reversal of expanded federal services and support for community mental health. The block grant that places responsibility for the delivery of mental health services at the state, rather than federal, level cannot help but have a profound effect on services delivery in the forthcoming decades. A complete appreciation of its impact requires that it be placed in context.

The Reagan Administration came into office on a philosophy that the federal government was the enemy; it had grown too large and powerful and was unresponsive to the needs of the people. Much of the social change wrought by the New Deal was suspect, and virtually all of the programs enacted in the past 20 years were targeted for modification or elimination. Health and human services programs would henceforth be the responsibility of the states. They would presumably be in a better position to determine needs and set priorities in these areas. We have argued that one of the failings of the community mental health program was the confusion resulting from the lack of direction and priorities at the federal level. It is difficult to see how moving responsibility for mental health to 50 different state mental health authorities or jurisdictions can improve the situation. If states do set priorities and goals consonant with local needs, we may have a situation in which intrastate homogeneity may be achieved at the expense of interstate or national coherence. The original goal of insuring that adequate mental health services are made available to all segments of the population without regard to race, socio-economic status, or geography will likely be lost. Although one could make the argument that the current decentralization provides an opportunity for constituency groups to operate on the state level to insure services for underserved populations, the lesson of history does not support this. Federal programs have come into being where state and local governments have not met health and human services needs.

It would be inaccurate to say that the Omnibus Reconciliation Act was a complete reversal of previous trends. One of the provisions of the Mental Health Systems Act called for a closer federal/state partnership to replace the federal/local relationship that had been operative under earlier legislation.

Although the report of the PCMH reiterated its support for the principle of community-based services, it also called for a more flexible and responsive system, one based on providing services consonant with local needs, rather than a set number. It seems likely that block grants will foster the continuation of this trend. Still, an obituary for community mental health seems premature. While federal support for the construction and staffing of CMHCs is at an end, the reality is that the program, in its 17 years of existence, did result in the establishment of over 700 centers. These centers, along with organizations like the National Council of Community Mental Health Centers, have become an established part of the mental health care delivery system and are unlikely to go away.

What does seem clearly at an end is the "mental health as panacea" ideology. It was unrealistic and unreasonable to expect that community mental health would solve all of society's problems. That it failed to do so was not surprising. There seems no likelihood that efforts at social activism and change will meet with much support. To equate social activism with community mental health would be an egregious error. The support of the PCMH for the principle of community-based mental health services was made in part on empirical evidence (e.g., Tischler et al., 1972) of the effectiveness of catchmenting in the delivery of mental health services. The public health model, then, does appear to be appropriate and is likely to be maintained.

This assertion has to be qualified, however, The withdrawal of federal support for mental health services raises serious questions about continued program direction. If states and localities take up the slack and mental health programs remain under public sponsorship, the public health model can likely be maintained. If, on the other hand, centers are increasingly forced to look to patient fees and third-party reimbursement for financial viability, the principle of catchmenting would appear to be imperiled.

Another trend likely to continue, one that antedates the Reagan Administration's policies, is mental health's (particularly psychiatry's) movement away from the social sciences. Psychiatry, after several decades as a quasi-social or behavioral science, is becoming more medical. Ozarin et al. (1979) have referred to this as the "mainstreaming of mental health into medicine." The de facto U.S. mental health system in which a majority of mental health care is rendered in the general medical sector (Regier et al., 1978) suggests that closer links should be forged between medicine and mental health. For some years, there have been federal programs to facilitate this linkage; the report of the PCMH called for this, and it was part of the Mental Health Systems Act.[5] Again, this trend is likely to continue, if not accelerate. There may be incentives for CMHCs to become more medical through additional third-party reimbursement. If mental health becomes more medical and less social, the continued viability of consultation and education programs and targeted prevention activities is problematic. In a positive sense, the "mainstreaming" of mental health into medicine may facilitate the delivery of services to the chronically ill and elderly, high-risk groups previously neglected by the mental health system.

We have just argued that the evidence for a closer link between health and mental health is strong. Another trend, one that is more difficult to document at this time, is an increasing use of institutional care for the mentally ill. If block grant monies are not used to support community programs at an adequate level, recourse to institutionalization may be necessary.

Some indirect support for this speculation may be found in some historical parallels. Levine and Levine's (1970) point made earlier, that political milieus generate different views of the locus of problems, may be instructive. In a liberal climate, social problems are seen as the result of defective social arrangements, and solutions involve social change. Conservative times, however, are likely to see social problems as the result of individual defects. Some measure of the conservative temper of the times may be gleaned from the administration's ban on social research and mental health. Henceforth, no funding will be forthcoming on the relationship between mental disorder and such social-structural variables as poverty, racism, or discrimination. This is obviously antipodal to the presumed etiological linkages between the social structure and mental disorder that were a cornerstone of the community mental health movement. If mental disorder is seen as some sort defect within the person, then hospitalization may be more easily seen as a solution. The Social Darwinism prevalent in the latter part of the last century that viewed the mentally ill as defectives and casualties of evolution helped to justify the rise of custodian hospitals.

On a less gothic level, Gerald Caplan, in an epilogue to Ruth Caplan's (1969) volume, has argued that interest in the relationship between community and mental health operates in terms of 20-year swings of a pendulum. The 1960s and 1970s were clearly periods of interest in the community. Now, with the 1980s, the pendulum is swinging away. This decreased interest in the community may facilitate the move toward institutions.

In sum, the community mental health movement must be seen as part of a long tradition of reform movements in U.S. history. It has had a substantial impact on the delivery of mental health services. Given the number of established CMHCs, it seems very likely to be a permanent feature of the health care system. Given the current fiscal restraints and conservative ideology in Washington, the exact form of community mental health in the coming decades is not entirely clear. We have, however, sketched out some possible directions.

Notes

1. Some controversy existed in this regard. Opponents argued that CMHCs established in general hospitals would likely be "swallowed up" in the general medical system (Lemkau, 1982).

2. See Coleman (Chapter 12, this volume) for more on the conceptual and empirical basis for this.

3. 1968 was the first year for which data were collected.

4. Lemkau (1982) has noted that the pattern of declining support for federal programs was modeled after the approach of some of the major foundations (e.g., Commonwealth, Rockefeller) in the health areas. Seed money would be used to demonstrate feasibility or effectiveness of an idea, and then local philanthropies or government would take over the operation. In the CMHC program, the transfer would be from the federal to the state level. In retrospect, the concept of declining federal fiscal participation may have been unrealistic, and some permanent base level of federal support should have been legislated.

5. For more on the relationship between health and mental health, see Coleman (Chapter 12, this volume).

References

ARNHOFF, F. D. Social consequences of policy toward mental illness. *Science*, 1975, *188*, 1277-1281.

BELLAK, L. Community psychiatry: The third psychiatric revolution. In L. Bellak (Ed.), *Handbook of community psychiatry and community mental health.* New York: Grune & Stratton, 1964.

BLOOM, B. L. *Community mental health.* Monterey, CA: Brooks/Cole, 1975.

BLUMER, H. Collective behavior. In A. M. Lee (Ed.), *Principles of sociology.* New York: Barnes & Noble, 1969.

BOCKOVEN, J. S. Community mental health: A new search for social orientation. *Psychiatric Opinion,* 1969, *6,* 4-13.

BURROWS, W. G. Community psychiatry–Another bandwagon? *Canadian Psychiatric Association Journal,* 1969, *14,* 105-114.

CAPLAN, R. B. *Psychiatry and the community in nineteenth century America.* New York: Basic Books, 1969.

CHU, F., & TROTTER, S. *The madness establishment.* New York: Grossman, 1973.

DEUTSCH, A. *The shame of the states.* New York: Harcourt Brace Jovanovich, 1948.

DINITZ, S., & BERAN, N. Community mental health as a boundaryless and boundary-busting system. *Journal of Health and Social Behavior,* 1971, *12,* 99-107.

DUNHAM, H. W. Community psychiatry: The newest therapeutic bandwagon. In J. Aronson (Ed.), *Current Issues in Psychiatry,* Vol. 1. New York: Science House, 1967.

EWALT, J. R., & EWALT, P. L. History of the community psychiatry movement. *American Journal of Psychiatry,* 1969, *126,* 43-52.

FELDMAN, S. Promises, promises, or community mental health services and training: Ships that pass in the night. *Community Mental Health Journal,* 1978, *14,* 83-91.

FELIX, R. H. Evolution of community mental health concepts. *American Journal of Psychiatry,* 1957, *114,* 673-679.

General Accounting Office. *Need for more effective management of the Community Mental Health Centers Program.* Report No. B-164031(5). Washington, DC: General Accounting Office, 1974.

HARRINGTON, M. *The other America.* New York: Penguin Books, 1962.

HEBERLE, R. *Social movements.* New York: Appleton-Century-Crofts, 1951.

HERSCH, C. Social history, mental health, and community control. *American Psychologist,* 1972, *27,* 749-754.

HOLLINGSHEAD, A. B., & REDLICH, F. C. *Social class and mental illness.* New York: John Wiley, 1958.

HUGHES, H. F. Emotional disturbance and American social change. *American Journal of Psychiatry,* 1969, *126,* 59-66.

Joint Commission on Mental Illness and Health. *Action for mental health.* New York: Basic Books, 1961.

JONES, M. *The maturation of the therapeutic community.* New York: Human Sciences Press, 1976.

KILLIAN, L. M., & TURNER, R. *Collective behavior* (2nd ed.) Englewood Cliffs, NJ: Prentice-Hall, 1972.

KOLB, L. C. Community mental health centers. *International Journal of Psychiatry,* 1970, *9,* 283-293.

LEIGHTON, A. H. *My name is legion.* New York: Basic Books, 1959.

LEMKAU, P. V. Personal communication, 1982.

LEVINE, M., & LEVINE, A. *A social history of helping services.* New York: Appleton-Century-Crofts, 1970.

MOYNIHAN, D. P. *Maximum feasible misunderstanding.* New York: Free Press, 1969.

MUSTO, D. Whatever happened to community mental health? *Public Interest,* 1975, *39,* 53-79.

OCHBERG, F. M., & OZARIN, L. D. The rationale of community mental health. Paper presented to the Kittay Scientific Foundation Symposium, New York, 1976.

OZARIN, L. D., SCHARFSTEIN, S. S., & ALBERT, M. Mainstreaming mental health into health. Paper presented to the annual meetings of the American Psychiatric Association, Chicago, 1979.

PANZETTA, A. *Community mental health–Myth and reality.* Philadelphia: Lea & Febiger, 1971.

PASAMANICK, B., SCARPITTI, F., & DINITZ, S. *Schizophrenics in the community.* New York: Appleton-Century-Crofts, 1967.

President's Commission on Mental Health. *Report to the President.* Washington, DC: Government Printing Office, 1978.

REGIER, D., GOLDBERG, I., & TAUBE, C. The de facto U.S. mental health services system. *Archives of General Psychiatry,* 1978, *35,* 685-696.

RIESSMAN, F., COHEN, J., & PEARL, A. (Eds.) *Mental health of the poor.* New York: Free Press, 1964.

ROSSI, A. M. Some pre-World War II antecedents of community mental health theory and practice. *Mental Hygiene,* 1962, *46,* 78-94.

SCHULBERG, H. C., & BAKER, F. Community mental health: The belief system of the 1960s. *Psychiatric Opinion,* 1969, *6,* 14-26.

SNOW, D., & NEWTON, P. Task, social structure and social process in the community mental health center movement. *American Psychologist,* 1976, *31,* 582-594.

SPANER, F. Personal communication, 1982.

SROLE, L., LANGNER, T. S., MICHAEL, S. T., OPLER, M. K., & RENNIE, T.A.C. *Mental health in the metropolis.* New York: McGraw-Hill, 1962.

TALBOT, J. A. Why psychiatrists leave the public sector. *Hospital and Community Psychiatry,* 1979, *30,* 778-782.

TISCHLER, G. L., HENISZ, J., MYERS, J. K., & GARRISON, V. The impact of catchmenting. *Administration in Mental Health,* 1972, Winter, 22-29.

USDHEW. *Community mental health centers–the federal investment.* Publication No. (ADM) 78-677. Rockville, MD: NIMH, 1978.

USDHHS. Annual inventory of comprehensive community mental health centers. Survey and Reports Branch, Division of Biometry and Epidemiology, NIMH. Unpublished data, 1980.

USDHHS. Office of Liaison and Program Analysis, Division of Mental Health Services Programs, NIMH. Unpublished data, 1981. (a)

USDHHS. *Toward a national plan for the chronically mentally ill.* Publication No. (ADM)81-1077, Washington, DC: Government Printing Office, 1981. (b)

WAGENFELD, M. O. The primary prevention of mental illness: A sociological perspective. *Journal of Health and Social Behavior,* 1972, *13,* 102-109.

WAGENFELD, M. O., & ROBIN, S. S. Social activism and community mental health: a policy perspective. *Administration in mental health,* 1980, *8,* 31-45.

WARREN, R. Types of purposive change at the community level. In R. Warren (Ed.), *Truth, love, and social change.* Chicago: Rand McNally, 1971.

WITKIN, M. J. *Trends in patient care episodes in mental health facilities.* Statistical Note 154, Survey and Reports Branch, Division of Biometry and Epidemiology. Rockville, MD: NIMH, 1980.

ZUSMAN, J., & LAMB, H. R. In defense of community mental health. *American Journal of Psychiatry,* 1977, *134,* 887-890.

Part II

ISSUES IN THE EPIDEMIOLOGY OF MENTAL DISORDERS

Chapter 4

RESEARCH PROGRESS 1955-1980

DARREL A. REGIER

This chapter will consider the accomplishments in mental health epidemiology of the past 25 years and reflect on its future objectives. Such an exercise might well begin by a review of the mental health field's historical context in 1955 (see Lemkau, Chapter 1; Ozarin, Chapter 2; and Wagenfeld & Jacobs, Chapter 3, this volume), followed by an assessment of how far we have come in meeting our expectations. Finally, we might briefly suggest some reasonable objectives for the future of our field which, in this chapter, will focus on mental health epidemiology research.

From an historical perspective, it might be observed that the field of psychiatric epidemiology at the start of our next quarter-century has many of the characteristics of the mid-1950s. Both the similarities and the differences should be instructive as we review our field in this presentation and in the others in this volume.

THE HISTORICAL CONTEXT OF MENTAL HEALTH EPIDEMIOLOGY

Epidemiological studies in the early 20th century had set the stage for much of the research that followed, from the mid-1950s to the present time. By 1920, Goldberger had shown that epidemiological investigations of pellagra-induced dementia could identify pathogenic dietary practices, the alteration of which lead to the prevention of the disorder (Terris, 1964). The correction of a nutritional deficiency, which was later shown to be niacin deficiency, resulted in the virtual disappearance of a disorder which was accounting for 10 percent of admissions to state mental hospitals in the Southern states (Cecil & Loeb, 1951: 575).

Following this public health triumph, Faris and Dunham (1939) used demographic mapping of mental hospital admissions in Chicago to show that higher rates of psychiatric hospitalization for schizophrenia were observed for persons coming from the inner-city areas. These areas were characterized as having high levels of social disorganization and social isolation—characteristics that were strikingly similar to the clinical description of schizophrenic patients. This study indicated that the social ecology of a patient's environment was associated with hospitalization for a severe psychiatric disorder. However, debates have continued to the present on whether social conditions caused the disorder or merely constituted a compatible environment into which persons with such disorders drifted.

World War II brought the problems of psychiatric disorders to public consciousness in a dramatic fashion. A number of studies showed that rates of psychiatric disorder for seemingly healthy soldiers varied in relation to the level of combat stress (Grinker & Spiegel, 1945). At the same time, large numbers of young men were never exposed to combat because of their rejection from military service for psychiatric reasons.

From these studies and others came the expectations that epidemiological research could be useful for studying the causes of mental disorders. A theoretical model of stress mediated through socioeconomic conditions or traumatic life experiences was postulated as possibly causing severe mental illnesses, and the large number of military recruit rejections led many to ask about the rate of mental disorders in the entire population.

The political context in 1955 was also right for supporting such research. The NIMH had been established in 1946 and was fully operational by 1949. A Joint Commission on Mental

Health (1961) was established in 1955, which was not unlike the recent President's Commission on Mental Health established in 1978. Finally, as a result of the establishment of both the NIMH and the Joint Commission, substantial support was available for determining the extent and nature of mental health problems in our society.

With this background in mind, we will now proceed to a review of epidemiological research from the past 25 years. As a structure for that review, we will use an outline of implied objectives provided by J. N. Morris (1957), who issued the first edition of his book entitled *The Uses of Epidemiology.* This book provides guidelines on how epidemiology can assist in reaching public health goals, and we can do well to check our performance against the potential functions or uses of epidemiology research. As a brief review, it should be recalled that these now well-known functions include the following: (1) documenting historical trends; (2) community diagnosis; (3) assessing the working of health services; (4) determining an individual's risks for developing illness; (5) completing the clinical picture by longitudinal studies of the natural history of an illness; (6) identifying new syndromes and illnesses; and (7) identifying causes to permit prevention of etiologically significant risk factors.

Before judging our performance to determine if we have been able to help the mental health field with these seven functions, it is important to recognize that several preconditions for good epidemiological research did not exist in 1955. Although some diagnostic consensus existed in the *Diagnostic and Statistical Manual* (DSM I) of the American Psychiatric Association (1952), for the definitions of most mental disorders, no reliable standardized procedure was available for assessing either patients or community residents to determine the presence of mental disorders. In fact, many analytically oriented U.S. psychiatrists tended to hold a unitary concept of mental illness that emphasized the etiological importance of intrapsychic conflicts for all mental disorders. Such disorders were seen as being on an uninterrupted symptomatic continuum with mental health (Menninger, 1963). The Adolph Meyer tradition, which emphasized the role of social and environmental stress in producing the "reactive disorders" of DSM I, also led to a cumulative stress model of mental disorder etiology. Diagnostic groups represented quantitative distinctions along a gradient rather than discrete, qualitatively separate entities with different genetic backgrounds, precipitants, or treatment responses. Hence, the epidemiological research efforts were limited by this significant theoretical framework, which included a bias toward viewing cumulative intrapsychic or sociocultural stresses as the most likely causative factors for mental disorders. Varying levels of stress could be seen as accounting for different degrees of mental disorder, ranging from normal, to neurotic, to psychotic.

THE SEARCH FOR CAUSES

Among the seven uses described by Morris, none was more vigorously pursued than the search for causes. By 1955, several large-scale epidemiological studies were already in progress, although the results would not be available for several years. The team of Alexander and Dorothea Leighton and colleagues had begun their study of Stirling County in an attempt to relate the level of community integration and disintegration to mental disorder levels (Leighton, 1959; Leighton et al., 1960). The hypothesis being tested was that socially disorganized and disintegrating communities both produce psychological dysfunction and simultaneously limit resources for dealing with it. To test this hypothesis, it was necessary to develop standardized measures of community status prior to conducting a community diagnosis of these theoretically independent and dependent variables. The methods used represented a significant advance in both survey design and diagnostic instrument development.

At about the same time, Thomas Rennie, Leo Srole, Thomas Langner, and their colleagues were analyzing data collected from a survey of Midtown Manhattan in 1953 (Srole et al., 1962). In this study, instead of measuring community disorganization, they developed a 10-factor measure of stress that included childhood economic deprivation, poor physical health, and poor interpersonal affiliations, among others. Hollingshead and Redlich (1958) were also completing the analysis of their 1950 study of New Haven psychiatric patients, which was reported in the 1958 publication of *Social Class and Mental Illness.* Although this was a treated prevalence rather than a true community prevalence survey, it was designed to look at differences in type, place, and length of psychiatric treatment in relationship to social class.

These three major studies of the early 1950s focused primarily on the social correlates of mental disorder and its treatment. They consistently showed a strong relationship between indicators of stress and reported rates of psychological disorder. The indicators of stress included community disorganization, a high multifactor stress score, and low socioeconomic status levels. However, the etiological significance of these findings is not yet clear. A large number of studies, including those by Eaton and Weil (1958), Clausen and Kohn (1959), Turner and Wagenfeld (1967), and others, attempted to determine whether the increased concentration of severe mental disorders in the lower socioeconomic levels was caused by the direct social consequences of living in poverty or was the more subtle, indirect result of social selection factors. Such factors include the possible downward socioeconomic drift of patients with mental disorders and their failure to rise from the social class of their parents at a normal rate.

Although the general population studies failed, by and large, to establish clear, preventable social risk factors, the association between indicators of stress (e.g., community disorganization) and risk of requiring mental health treatment were important from the mental health services policy perspective. If social factors within the community cause mental disorders, both preventive and therapeutic interventions could be focused more effectively if services were provided within a well-defined community or geographical area. The resultant epidemiologically based theoretical framework helped launch the Community Mental Health Center Program with its emphasis on community locus of treatment, community board participation, and consultation/education prevention efforts.

The designation of catchment areas or denominator populations could have facilitated determinations of mental disorder rates within the catchment areas, followed by assessments of how therapeutic and preventive services affected these rates. However, it is not clear that an epidemiology of specific mental disorders would have been seen as necessary, even if the technology for such an effort had been available. It was assumed that there was more mental disorder in the community than could be treated, and the major goal was to increase mental health service use—an accomplishment that the catchmenting method and the general increase in supply of services certainly accomplished (Taube et al., 1978: ch. 4).

The true nature of the association between community socioeconomic variables, other stress-related variables, and mental disorders was not elucidated by the natural experiment of introducing treatment and prevention services into CMHC catchment areas. Failure to have pre- and postservice prevalence and incidence rates, as well as the absence of clearly defined risk factor studies, made the testing of this association impossible.

Following the striking scientific discoveries in psychopharmacology of chlorpromazine, tricyclic antidepressants, and lithium, together with the neurobiological discoveries of chemical brain neurotransmitters affected by these drugs, interest in the biological and genetic factors that might cause the serious mental disorders was substantially increased. Seymour Kety and his colleagues (1968) conducted an elegant case-control study that determined the relative risk of schizophrenia among biological and adoptive relatives of persons with schizophrenia.

This research was conducted by applying epidemiologic methods to genetically defined populations in order to establish convincingly that the risk of developing schizophrenia is substantially increased by genetic transmission. Ming Tsuang and George Winokur (1975) have also shown a pronounced tendency of major affective disorders to develop via genetic transmission.

However, biological models that explain the greater risk for mental disorder in family members with a positive genetic background do not yet offer adequate scientific frameworks for a complete understanding of the etiology of mental disorders. Likewise, an exclusive focus on sociocultural factors has not led to a comprehensive understanding or documented prevention of any of the major mental disorders.

What appears to be needed is a multifactorial approach that considers both environmental (stress) factors and host (biological or personality) factors as independent variables contributing to a mental disorder's development. Improvements in the specification of these independent variables and the diagnostic, dependent variables will make risk factor reasearch increasingly possible (Regier & Allen, 1981).

COMMUNITY DIAGNOSIS

In the area of community diagnosis, both the Sterling County and the Midtown Manhattan studies found serious impairment in over 20 percent of the population. However, the impact of informing the public that only 15 percent of the population in Midtown Manhattan could be considered completely well led many to insist on more precise definitions of what constitutes mental disorder. A more conservative diagnostic-specific survey was performed by Pasamanick et al. (1956) in Baltimore, who found about 10 percent of the population with specific diagnosable mental disorders. Because of the use of physicians to both screen and verify the presence of specific psychiatric disorders, this rigorous study has been used as a conservative U.S. standard (Regier et al., 1978).

There have also been a considerable number of important epidemiological studies of general practitioners' patients (Hankin & Oktay, 1979). This interest is partially due to the fact that a large portion of the general population uses such physicians in one year; hence, general practitioners can assist in the case identification of noninstitutionalized persons with mental disorders. Michael Shepherd et al. (1966) produced a major study of this type in England and found rates of about 14 percent with mental disorders in one year. Similar studies by Locke and Gardner (1969) and Rosen et al. (1972) in the United States found comparable rates. However, no national estimates of the prevalence or incidence of specific mental disorders yet exist in this or any other country.

WORKING OF HEALTH SERVICES

In addition to community diagnosis functions, treatment implications for patients with identified mental disorders may be assessed in general practice studies as part of our examination of the third element of Morris's system—the workings of the health care system. In a recent publication for the President's Commission on Mental Health, staff from our division were able to show that the majority of patients with mental disorders rely heavily on the general medical sector for mental health care (Regier et al., 1978). Using the conservative 15 percent estimate of mental disorder prevalence in the community, it was possible through secondary data analyses to determine that psychiatrists and other mental health professionals were able to see only 3 percent of the population per year. This represents some 20 percent of those with identifiable mental disorders. Fully 54 percent of such persons were seen to rely exclusively on the primary care outpatient sector, with an additional 3 percent seen in nursing homes or general hospitals. These findings, noted in the President's Commission on Mental Health Report, had potential service policy implications, as reflected in the Mental Health Systems Act's emphasis on integrating health and mental health services (PL 96-398, 1980).

HISTORICAL TRENDS

In the area of historical trends, we have been able to follow the epidemiology of health service use somewhat better than the epidemiology of mental health status. We have been able to document historical trends in the changing locus of treatment for patients with mental disorders from state mental hospitals out into community-based settings. The changes in year-end censuses of state and county mental hospitals from a 1955 high of over 550,000 to the present level of about 140,000 document a major trend in the epidemiology of mental health service use (Regier & Taube, 1980).

Although some of the unintended consequences of deinstitutionalization are now being grappled with, the availability of these and more complex service use data, collected by the NIMH under Morton Kramer's direction for most of the 25 years we are reviewing, has added immeasurably to our ability to document changes and define our problems.

DETERMINING INDIVIDUAL RISKS

There are only two other uses by Morris that I will review before looking briefly to the future. They include the determination of individual risks and identifying syndromes.

As a result of work by Kety and Winokur, individual risks of developing schizophrenia, manic depressive or bipolar affective illness, or severe unipolar depressive disorders may now be determined if one knows a person's genetic history for these disorders. Holmes and Rahe (1967) have also increased our sophistication in predicting the onset of either physical or mental disorders from scores on life event stress scales. The prediction of the lifetime use of mental health services from both case register life table analysis methods and from the longitudinal studies of Hagnell (1966) also constitute significant contributions to the field.

In the identification of syndromes or new disease entities, there have been substantial improvements in the diagnostic systems leading to the Spitzer et al. (1978) Research Diagnostic Criteria (RDC) and to the *Diagnostic and Statistical Manual of Mental Disorders* (DSM III) of the American Psychiatric Association (1980), both operational definitions of mental disorders (Feighner et al., 1972). However, clinical and not epidemiological studies contributed most to these developments. An important contribution in this area was made by Ernest Gruenberg (1974: 697-711), whose careful observations of the secondary consequences of institutionalization led to the identification of the social breakdown syndrome, which could be prevented by careful attention to maintaining patient community contacts and preventing institutional depersonalization. This finding can be linked in part to previous sociological research by Goffman (1961), who identified the characteristics of residents living in a wide range of total institutions.

In summary, our scorecard in translating epidemiological research into useful public health applications is still somewhat modest. However, the major limiting factor for epidemiological research in this field has been the lack of rigorous diagnostic criteria for mental disorders and a suitable case-finding instrument that could be reliably applied in both community and clinical settings. As in all of epidemiology, if you can't define a specific illness or identify it readily with reliable and valid techniques, it is rather difficult to correlate the dependent variable (mental disorder conditions) with independent risk factor variables that might offer causative explanations.

THE FUTURE

Despite this somewhat sober assessment of the field, I believe that the past contributions of psychiatric epidemiology provide a firm basis for higher expectations in the future. The U.S.-U.K. study demonstrated that two countries, using general criteria from the International Classification of Diseases, could have wide differences in reported hospital admission rates for schizophrenia and affective illnesses (Cooper et al., 1972). When more refined diagnostic criteria were used, the differences disappeared. The *International Pilot Study of Schizophrenia* (IPSS) of WHO extended the U.S.-U.K. methodology by demonstrating that schizophrenia, defined by rigorous criteria, can be found in multiple countries with widely different sociodemographic and genetic characteristics (World Health Organization, 1973).

With the development of the Research Diagnostic Criteria and the *DSM-III* standardized classification, observable and operational criteria for diagnosis of the full range of mental disorders are now available. The development of standardized psychiatric interviews, such as the NIMH *Diagnostic Interview Schedule* (DIS) (Robins et al., 1978; Robins et al., 1981) should facilitate a new generation of improved epidemiological research studies. Of immediate relevance are the NIMH Epidemiologic Catchment Area (ECA) studies in several U.S. communities (Eaton et al., 1981). These studies will link prevalence and incidence rates in both institutionalized and community populations. In addition, data on the presence of a mental disorder will be related to longitudinal health service utilization information to assist us in fulfilling a number of Morris's uses of epidemiology.

It should be noted that there are several interesting parallels between 1955 and 1980 in the epidemiological research field. The President's Commission on Mental Health has reemphasized the need for specific diagnostic data on the prevalence of persons with mental disorders and on the workings of the health system to meet their needs. Funding has become available to support the first large-scale epidemiological studies in almost 20 years. At the present time, five Epidemiologic Catchment Area programs under NIMH sponsorship are now underway to provide such information using the NIMH-DIS case-finding instrument.

Finally, a theoretical framework now exists that considers the etiological importance of both biological and sociocultural factors. This balanced approach offers new opportunities for discovering a causal chain for specific disorders which, if broken, may lead to better prevention opportunities. The linking of information on the presence of a mental disorder with data on a patient's use of specialty mental health, general medical, and other human services will greatly assist in both planning and assessing the workings of the health system. Longitudinal follow-up studies should provide additional information on the natural course of these clearly defined disorders. Finally, the application of standardized methods should allow for future applications in multiple sites to permit historical trend determinations of changes in mental disorder prevalence and incidence rates associated with changes in either the environment or in our treatment and prevention efforts.

References

American Psychiatric Association. *Diagnostic and statistical manual of mental disorders* (1st ed.) Washington, DC: Author, 1952.

American Psychiatric Association. *Diagnostic and statistical manual of mental disorders* (3rd ed.) Washington, DC: Author, 1980.

CECIL, R. L., & LOEB, R. F. *Textbook of medicine* (8th ed.) Philadelphia: W. B. Saunders, 1951.

CLAUSEN, J. A., & KOHN, M. L. Relation of schizophrenia to the social structure of a small city. *Epidemiology of mental disorder.* Washington, DC: American Association for the Advancement of Science, 1959.

COOPER, J. E., KENDELL, R. E., GURLAND, B. J., SHARPE, L., COPELAND, J.R.M., & SIMON, R. *Psychiatric diagnosis in New York and London.* London: Oxford University Press, 1972.

EAT& WEIL, R. J. *Culture and mental disorders.* New York: Free Press, 1955.

EATON, W. W., REGIER, D. A., LOCKE, B. Z., & TAUBE, C. A. The NIMH epidemiologic catchment area program. *Public Health Reports,* 1981, *96,* No. 4.

FARIS, R.E.L., & DUNHAM, H. W. *Mental disorders in urban areas: An ecological study of schizophrenia and other psychoses.* Chicago: The University of Chicago Press, 1939.

FEIGHNER, J. P., ROBINS, E., & GUZE, S. B. Diagnostic criteria for use in psychiatric research. *Archives of General Psychiatry,* 1972, *26,* 57-63.

GOFFMAN, E. Essays on the social situation of mental patients and other inmates. In *Asylums.* Chicago: Aldine, 1961.

GRINKER, R. R., & SPIEGEL, J. P. *Men under stress.* Philadelphia: Blakiston, 1945.

GRUENBERG, E. M. The social breakdown system and its prevention. In G. Caplan (Ed.), *American Handbook of Psychiatry* (2nd ed.), Vol. II: Child and adolescent psychiatry, sociocultural and community psychiatry. New York: Basic Books, 1974.

HAGNELL, O. *A prospective study of the incidence of mental disorder.* Sweden: Scandinavian University Books, 1966.

HANKIN, J., & OKTAY, J. S. *Mental disorder and primary medical care: An analytical review of the literature.* DHEW Publication No. ADM-78-661. Washington, DC: Government Printing Office, 1979.

HOLLINGSHEAD, A. B., & REDLICH, F. D. *Social class and mental illness.* New York: John Wiley, 1958.

HOLMES, T. H., & RAHE, R. H. The social readjustment rating scale. *Journal of Psychosomatic Research,* 1967, *11,* 213-218.

Joint Commission on Mental Illness and Health. *Action for mental health.* New York: Basic Books, 1961.

KETY, S. S., ROSENTHAL, D., WENDER, P. H., & SCHULSINGER, F. The types and prevalence of mental illness in the biological and adoptive families of adopted schizophrenics. In D. Rosenthal & S. S. Kety (Eds.), *The transmission of schizophrenia.* London: Pergamon Press, 1968.

LEIGHTON, A. H. *My name is legion.* New York: Basic Books, 1959.

LEIGHTON, D. C., HARDING, J. S., & MACKLIN, D. R. *The character of danger.* New York: Basic Books, 1960.

LOCKE, B. Z., & GARDNER, E. Psychiatric disorders among the patients of general practitioners and internists. *Public Health Reports,* 1969, *84,* 167-173.

MENNINGER, K. *The vital balance.* New York: Viking Press, 1963.

MORRIS, J. N. *The uses of epidemiology.* London: E. & S. Livingstone, 1957.

PASAMANICK, B., ROBERTS, D. W., & LEMKAU, P. V. A survey of mental disease in an urban population. *American Journal of Public Health,* 1956, *47,* 923-929.

The President's Commission on Mental Health. *Report to the President.* Washington, DC: Government Printing Office, 1978.

REGIER, D. A., & ALLEN, G. (Eds.) *Risk factor research in the major mental disorders.* DHHS Publication No. (ADM) 81-1068. Washington, DC: Government Printing Office, 1981.

REGIER, D. A., & TAUBE, C. A. The delivery of mental health services—where and by whom. In *American handbook of psychiatry* (2nd ed.), Vol. VII. New York: Basic Books, 1980.

REGIER, D. A., GOLDBERG, I. G., & TAUBE, C. A. The de facto U.S. mental health services system: A public health perspective. *Archives of General Psychiatry,* 1978, *35,* 685-693.

ROBINS, L. N., HELZER, J. H., CROUGHAN, J., & RATCLIFF, K. S. National Institute of Mental Health diagnostic interview schedule: Its history, characteristics, and validity. *Archives of General Psychiatry,* 1981, *38,* 381-389.

ROBINS, L. N., HELZER, J. H., CROUGHAN, J., WILLIAMS, J.B.W., & SPITZER, R. L. *The NIMH diagnostic interview schedule.* Rockville, MD: NIMH, 1978.

ROSEN, B. M., LOCKE, B. Z., & GOLDBERG, I. D. Identification of emotional disturbance in patients seen in general medical clinics. *Hospital & Community Psychiatry,* 1972, *23,* 364-370.

SHEPHERD, M., COOPER, B., BROWN, A. C., & KALTON, G. W. *Psychiatric illness in general practice.* London: Oxford University Press, 1966.

SPITZER, R. L., ENDICOTT, J., & ROBINS, E. Research diagnostic criteria. *Archives of General Psychiatry,* 1978, *35,* 773-782.

SROLE, L., LANGNER, T. S., & MACKLIN, D. B. *Mental health in the metropolis: The Midtown Manhattan study.* New York: McGraw-Hill, 1962.

TAUBE, C. A., REGIER, D. A., & ROSENFELD, A. H. Mental disorders. In *Health, United States, 1978.* DHEW Publication No. (PHS) 78-1232. Washington, DC: Government Printing Office, 1978.

TERRIS, M. (Ed.) *Goldberger on pellagra.* Baton Rouge: Louisiana State University Press, 1964.

TISCHLER, G. L., HENISZ, J., MYERS, J. K. & GARRISON, V. Catchmenting and the use of mental health services. *Archives of General Psychiatry,* 1972, *27,* 389-392.

TSUANG, M. T., & WINOKUR, G. The Iowa 500: Fieldwork in a 35-year followup of depression, mania, and schizophrenia. *Journal of the Canadian Psychiatric Association,* 1975, *20,* 359-365.

TURNER, R., & WAGENFELD, M. Occupational mobility and schizophrenia: An assessment of social causation and social selection hypothesis. *American Sociological Review,* 1967, *32,* 104-113.

World Health Organization. *The international pilot study of schizophrenia,* Vol. 1. Geneva: Author, 1973.

Chapter 5

THE CONTINUING CHALLENGE
The Rising Prevalence of Mental Disorders, Associated Chronic Diseases, and Disabling Conditions

MORTON KRAMER

Despite the accomplishments of the past 25 years, we still have major problems to solve if we are to make further progress in our efforts to reduce the prevalence of mental disorders and chronic diseases and the disabling conditions associated with them.

To emphasize this point, I propose to look ahead to the year 2005 to provide some idea of the magnitude of the problem of the mental disorders and associated chronic diseases and disabling conditions that will be confronting us in the next 25 years. In doing this, I have paid particular attention to that section of the report of the President's Commission on Mental Health (1978: 49) which underscored the urgent need for epidemiological data on the mental disorders, data on utilization of health and mental health services by persons with these disorders, and related socioeconomic and demographic data. The commission stated:

> Long-term epidemiological and survey research are necessary in order to understand the incidence and scope of mental disorders in this country. The need for more precise demographic and socioeconomic data is urgent if we are to understand and meet the different needs which exist in our society. Data to determine the availability and utilization of services are also insufficient. Without such data it is difficult to assess needs or to plan for and deliver services. The Commission therefore recommends:
>
> Immediate efforts to gather reliable data (including socioeconomic and demographic data) on the incidence of mental health problems and the utilization of mental health services. Particular attention should be paid to population groups within our society known to have special needs, such as children, adolescents, the aging, women, and racial and ethnic minorities.
>
> Increased research efforts designed to produce greater understanding of the needs and problems of people who are underserved or inappropriately served or who are at high risk for mental disorders.

HOW I HAVE LOOKED AHEAD

I have approached the problem of projecting numbers of persons with mental disorders and related conditions by asking the following question: Suppose the incidence and prevalence rates of specific mental disorders by age, sex, and race are the same in the year 2005 as they are in the year 1980. How many cases of mental disorders would we have in the year 2005? What would the total (crude) prevalence rates be? Higher or lower than in 1980? Stated differently, despite all of our efforts, we will not have been able to lower prevalence rates by the time the Mental Health Section of the American Public Health Association will celebrate its 50th anniversary. If this is the case, then, assuming a 15 percent prevalence rate of all disorders (Regier et al., 1978), the number of persons with mental disorders will increase from 33,323,850 in 1980 to 40,140,300 in 2005, an overall increase of 20.0 percent. Among the white population, the number will increase from 28,737,150 in 1980 to 33,777,900 in 2005, an increase of 18 percent. Among black and other races, the increase will be from 4,586,700 to 6,362,400, an increase of 39 percent, and more than twice that for the white population.[1] These increases will be brought about merely by the following expected increases in population during the next quarter-century as shown in Table 5.1 (U.S. Bureau of the Census, 1977a).

The above computations emphasize that if there is no change in total prevalence rates and these rates remain at the 1980 level for whites and nonwhites, then the relative increase in the number of cases will be the same as the relative increase in the general population. I wish to underscore this simple but basic point, which is often overlooked but must be kept in mind. However, the above computations do not take into account changes in the age-sex-race distribution of the population nor in the incidence and prevalence rates of mental disorders specific for these factors.

Although estimates of the population of the United States and their projections are available by age, sex, and race, corresponding estimates and projections are not available for the prevalence and incidence rates of mental disorders. To prepare this chapter, I had to find proxies for these rates and then ask the question stated above: namely, if the rates for various conditions selected show no change between 1980 and 2005, what will be the number of cases that we would have in 2005, specific for age-race-sex and for various combinations of these variables? What would be the total (crude) prevalence rates?

I believe this approach is reasonable yet conservative for the following reasons. Unless some unexpected breakthroughs occur that provide us with the knowledge needed to prevent the occurrence of specific mental disorders and, equally important, the methods to apply this knowledge effectively, it is highly unlikely that we will witness any significant decline in their incidence rates. The group of mental disorders I am referring to includes various organic psychotic conditions (e.g., senile dementia–Alzheimer's type, multi-infarct dementias, alcoholic and toxic psychoses); other psychoses (schizophrenia and affective psychoses); and various neurotic and personality disorders.

On the other hand, we will certainly witness an increase in prevalence. Remember the basic epidemiologic relationship:

The prevalence of a disorder varies as the product of its incidence and its duration. The duration of most disorders will increase. The reason is that the newer treatment methods for various mental disorders and advances in psychiatric, medical, and social care, which ameliorate and/or control these conditions and arrest their fatal complications, have prolonged the lives of affected individuals. Thus, in the absence of effective measures for reducing incidence, prevalence will increase.

In "Failures of Success," Gruenberg (1977) commented as follows on the increase in age-specific prevalence rates:

> It is obvious that, with increasing duration, we would expect the proportion of the population in any given age group suffering from these conditions to rise. And, in fact, as the result of advances in medical care, we are seeing a rising prevalence of certain chronic conditions which previously led to early terminal infections, but whose victims now suffer from them for a longer period. The goal of medical research work is to "diminish disease and enrich life" (Gregg, 1941), but it produced tools which prolong diseased, diminished lives and so increased the proportion of people who have a disabling or chronic disease.
>
> That is a major but unintended effect of many technical improvements stemming from health research. These increasingly common chronic conditions represent the failures of success. Their growing prevalence and longer duration are a product of progress in health technology.

In addition to the role being played by technical improvements in medical and psychiatric care, another phenomenon is operating that will add significantly to the prevalence count. Large relative increases are occurring in numbers of persons in age groups at high risk for developing mental disorders and associated chronic diseases and disabling conditions. This phenomenon increases total (crude) prevalence rates. As a result of the simultaneous operation of two forces–one, increasing age-specific prevalence rates, and the other, large relative increases in the number of persons in high-risk groups–prevalence is bound to increase.

SOURCES OF DATA

What data are needed to answer the question posed earlier concerning the incidence and prevalence of mental disorders and associated conditions in 2005? Two types of data are needed: incidence and prevalence rates by age, race, and sex for mental disorders as a group and for specific disorders within the group, and population estimates specific for age, sex, and race for 1980 and for the projected populations of the year 2005.

As Finagle (in Carruthers et al., 1972) once said in his three laws of information: The information you have is not that which you want; the information you want is not that which you need; the information you need is not that which you can obtain. To which I add: Make the most out of that which is available.

POPULATION PROJECTIONS

With respect to the population projections, I am using those prepared by the U.S. Bureau of the Census (1977a) by age, sex, and race for the United States from 1977 to the year 2005. The Bureau of the Census presented three different series of estimates based on ultimate levels of cohort fertility (average number of lifetime births per woman), various assumptions about mortality that reflect the recent decline in age-specific death rates in the middle and older adult ages, and recent research on future trends in mortality and an assumed constant level of net immigration of 400,000 persons per year. Time does not permit discussion of these various assumptions, but those interested should read the detailed discussions provided by the U.S. Bureau of the Census (1977a). For purposes of this chapter I have used the series II projections, which assume an average of 2.1 lifetime births per woman. These are essentially the "middle" projections.

The population estimates for 1980, the projections for 2005, and the expected percentage increases in number are given by age for the white and nonwhite populations in Table 5.1 and Figure 5.1.

Table 5.1 Population (in thousands) by Age Group, Sex, and Race, Projected from 1980[a] to 2005[b]

Age Group (Years)	1980	2005	% Change	1980	2005	% Change
	WHITES			BLACK AND OTHER		
			BOTH SEXES			
Total	191,581	225,186	17.5	30,578	42,416	38.7
15	41,220	45,804	11.1	8,696	9,840	13.2
15-24	35,027	32,517	- 7.2	6,499	7,508	15.5
25-34	31,254	27,196	-13.0	4,919	6,207	26.2
35-44	22,464	32,402	44.2	3,256	5,996	84.2
45-54	19,956	33,897	69.9	2,743	5,485	99.9
55-64	19,078	24,662	29.3	2,120	3,653	72.3
65-74	13,945	15,176	8.8	1,548	2,209	42.7
75 +	8,634	13,532	56.7	797	1,518	90.5
			MALES			
Total	93,621	109,926	17.4	14,600	20,110	37.7
15	21,112	23,510	11.4	4,392	5,011	14.1
15-24	17,769	16,560	- 6.8	3,218	3,772	17.2
25-34	15,714	13,688	-12.9	2,279	2,944	29.2
35-44	11,090	16,077	44.9	1,470	2,720	85.0
45-54	9,758	16,725	71.4	1,271	2,497	96.5
55-64	9,065	11,950	31.8	975	1,659	70.2
65-74	6,038	6,718	11.3	675	945	40.0
75 +	3,075	4,698	52.8	320	562	75.6
			FEMALES			
Total	97,957	115,260	17.7	15,978	22,306	39.6
15	20,108	22,294	10.9	4,304	4,829	12.2
15-24	17,258	15,957	- 7.5	3,281	3,736	13.9
25-34	15,540	13,508	-13.1	2,640	3,263	23.6
35-44	11,374	16,325	43.6	1,786	3,276	83.4
45-54	10,198	17,172	68.4	1,472	2,988	102.9
55-64	10,013	12,712	27.0	1,145	1,994	74.2
65-74	7,907	8,458	7.0	873	1,264	44.8
75 +	5,559	8,834	58.9	477	956	100.4

a. U.S. Bureau of the Census. *Projections of the population of the United States, 1977-2050. Current Population Reports,* Series P-25, No. 704 (Table 8), 1977.

b. U.S. Bureau of the Census. The bureau provided the projected population (Series II) for 2005 by age and sex only. The age, sex, and race distribution for 2005 was prepared under the assumption that the corresponding distributions for the year 2000 applied to the estimated 2005 age-sex distribution.

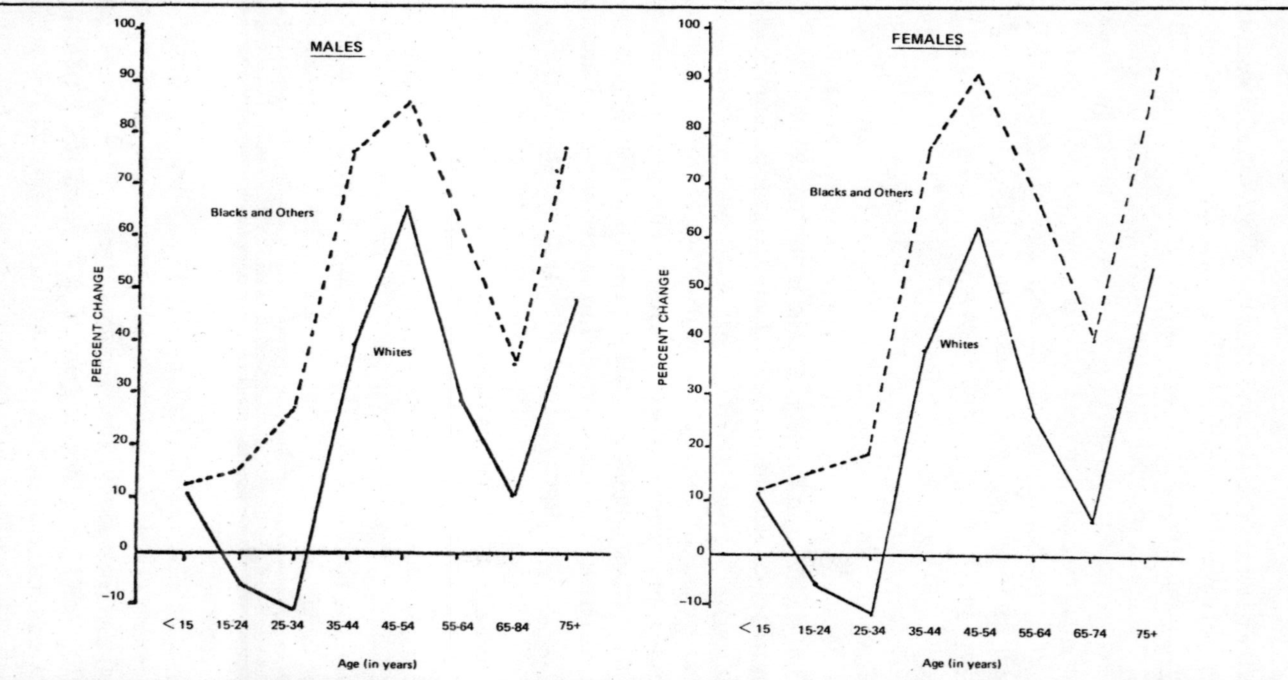

Figure 5.1 Percentage Change in the U.S. Population, 1980-2005

SOURCE: Bureau of the Census. **Projections of the population of the United States, 1977-2050.** Current Population Reports, Series P-25, No. 704, 1977.

Note that in the "black and other races" group, the relative increases between 1980 and 2005 exceed the corresponding increases among whites by a substantial amount in 7 out of the 8 age groups. The exception is the under-15-years age group, where the percentage increase is only slightly higher for blacks and other races (13 percent) than for whites (11 percent). Whites are expected to experience decreases in persons in the 15-24 and 25-34 age groups. Persons who will be under 25 years in 2005 are yet to be born, and the uncertain level of the birth rates in the next two decades makes projections for these age groups quite uncertain. The decrease in persons 25-34 years results from the decreases in white births that occurred during the past decade. Currently, the birth rate is starting to increase slowly, but its trend in the next decade is still uncertain.

The number of persons in each of the age groups from 35-44 years through 75 years and over will increase both for whites and other races, but the relative increase for the other races is considerably in excess of that for whites. This phenomenon is due to the remarkable gains made during this century by members of this group in their survivorship to the age of 65 and to the increase in the expectation of life for those who survive to this age (Table 5.2). For example, during the years 1900-1902, the percentage of all other races surviving to age 65 was 22 percent for females and 19 percent for males. By 1977, corresponding figures were 73 percent for females (230 percent increase) and 55.8 percent for males (193 percent increase). For the white population in 1900-1902, the percentage of females surviving to age 65 was 43.8 percent and males 39.2 percent. By 1977, the corresponding figures rose to 83.8 percent for females (an increase of 91 percent) and 70.7 percent for males (an 80 percent increase).

There were also remarkable gains in the expectation of life at age 65 years (Table 5.2). For blacks and other races, these expectations increased for females from 11.4 years in 1900-1902 to 17.8 years, a gain of 6.4 years (56.1 percent increase) and for males, from 10.4 to 14.0, a gain of 3.6 years (34.6 percent increase). For the white population, the corresponding increase for females was from 12.2 years to 18.4 years, a gain of 6.2 years (50.8 percent increase) and for males from

Table 5.2 Percentage Surviving from Birth to Age 65 and Expectation of Life Beyond Age 65, By Race and Sex: Death Registration States, 1900-1902, and United States, 1959-1971 and 1977[a]

YEAR	Total	WHITE Male	WHITE Female	ALL OTHER Male	ALL OTHER Female
	Percentage Surviving from Birth to Age 65				
1977	75.8	70.7	83.8	55.8	72.7
1969-71	71.9	66.3	81.6	49.6	66.1
1959-61	71.1	65.8	80.7	51.4	60.8
1900-1902	40.9	39.2	43.8	19.0	22.0
	Expectation of Life Beyond Age 65 (in years)				
1977	16.3	13.9	18.4	14.0	17.8
1969-71	15.00	13.02	16.93	12.87	15.99
1959-61	14.39	12.97	15.88	12.84	15.12
1900-1902	11.86	11.51	12.23	10.38	11.38

SOURCE: National Center for Health Statistics. *Vital Statistics of the United States, 1977,* Vol. II. *Life tables.* DHEW Publication No. (PHS)80-1104. Washington, DC: Author, 1980.

a. For 1900-1902, figures for "all other male" and "all other female" include only the black population, which comprised 95 percent or more of the "all other" population.

11.5 years to 13.9 years, a gain of 2.4 years (20.9 percent increase).

MORBIDITY AND OTHER DATA

The lack of data on incidence and prevalence rates for various mental disorders posed problems. Systematic annual morbidity rates on mental disorders specific for age, sex, race, and diagnosis are not available for the United States and its various subdivisions, or for that matter for any other country of the world.

For puposes of this chapter, the age-specific treated incidence and prevalence rates for schizophrenia, derived from the psychiatric case register for Monroe County, New York, were used (Babigian, 1975). These are shown in Figure 5.2. Those for senile dementia were derived from studies done in Lund, Sweden (Hagnell & Gruenberg, 1978). In the opinion of experts in these fields, the shapes of the age-specific curves for these conditions as reported in these studies are likely to be the same

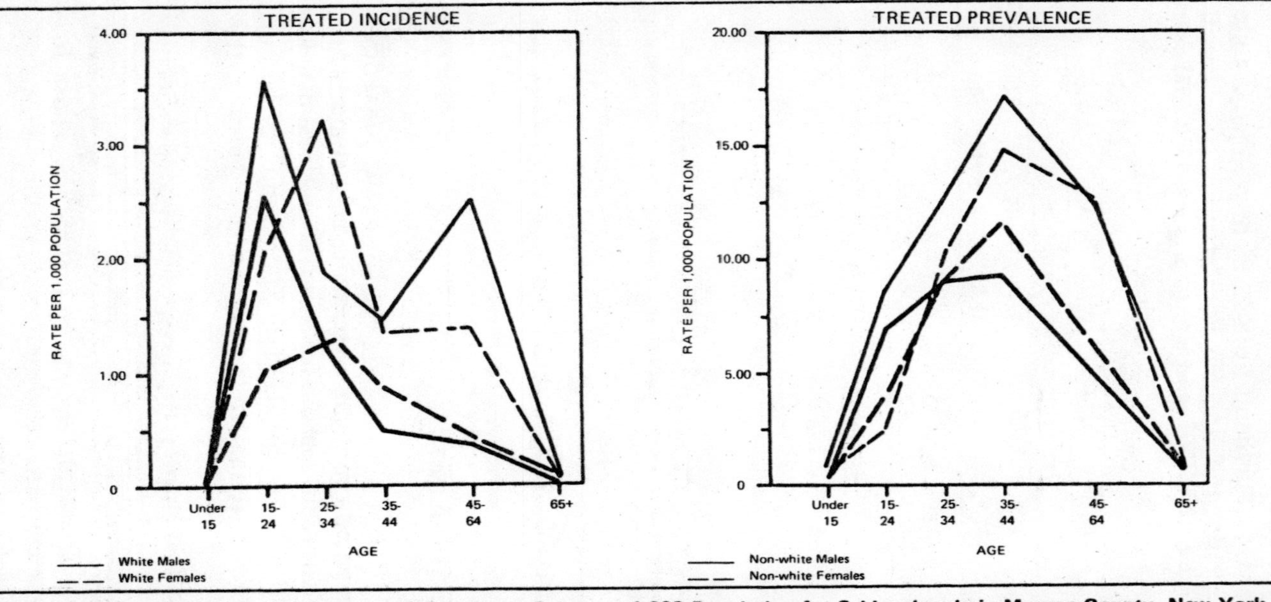

Figure 5.2 Age-Specific Treated Incidence and Prevalence Rates per 1,000 Population for Schizophrenia in Monroe County, New York, by Race and Sex, 1970

Treated Incidence = Number of new cases of schizophrenia (hospitalized and not hospitalized) reported to Monroe County Case Register during the calendar year 1970, per 1,000 population.

Treated Prevalence = Number of cases of schizophrenia (hospitalized and not hospitalized) known to have received care during 1970, per 1,000 population.

SOURCE: Based on Figures from H. M. Babigian, Schizophrenia: Epidemiology. In A. M. Freedman and B. J. Sadock (Eds.), **Comprehensive textbook of psychiatry, Vol. II.** Baltimore, MD: Williams & Wilkins, 1975.

from country to country, but their levels—that is, the absolute numerical values of the rates—may vary. However, their actual levels will not be known until the data needed to determine them become available.

Three other types of data were used: (1) admission rates to all psychiatric facilities for the year 1975, prepared by the NIMH Division of Biometry and Epidemiology from their national reporting program (National Institute of Mental Health, 1981a) (see Figure 5.3); (2) resident patient rates of nursing homes derived from the Survey of Nursing Homes of the National Center for Health Statistics (1977) (see Figure 5.4); and (3) age-, sex-, and race-specific mortality rates for selected diagnoses, prepared by the National Center for Health Statistics (1979).

The mortality rates slected were those that provide indicators of diseases and conditions of concern to the mental health field. Rates specific for age, sex, and race for the following causes of death in the year 1975 were used (NCHS, 1979): cerebrovascular disease (A85),[2] cirrhosis of the liver (A102), suicides (AE147), motor vehicle accidents (AE138), all other accidents (A139-146), and homicides (AE148).[3]

Deaths from these conditions represent the end result of underlying diseases or conditions that are frequently associated with mental disorder: brain syndromes associated with cerebrovascular disease; alcoholism that results in liver cirrhosis; depressive and other disorders associated with suicide; psychological and behavioral factors associated with motor vehicle accidents, as well as the large number of head injuries, skull fractures, and emotional upsets that appear in persons involved in such accidents; psychological, emotional, and other problems associated with other accidents that happen to people in every age group; and the violent and other antisocial attitudes that lead to homicide. Thus, high mortality rates for these disorders are indicators of high underlying morbidity rates for various associated types of mental disorders.

The above causes appear among the 5-10 leading causes of death among various age groups. Accordingly, not only the health but the mental health and social problems represented by

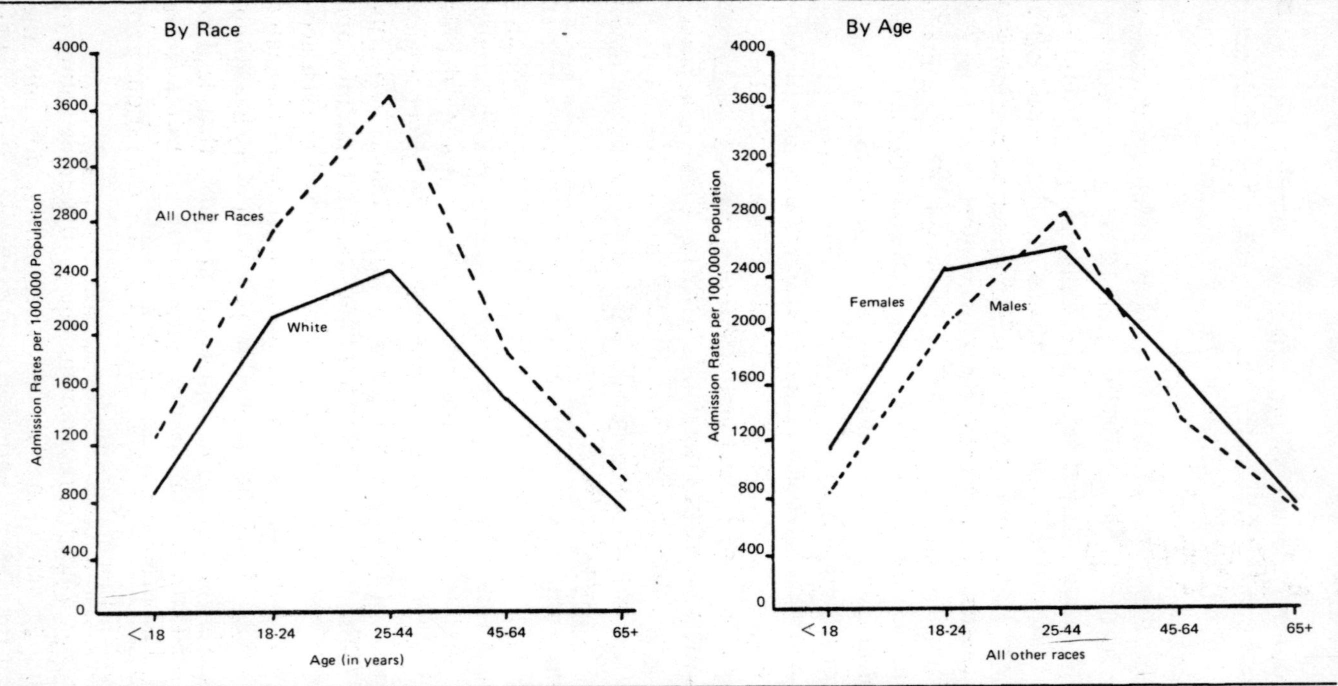

Figure 5.3 Admission Rates per 1,000 Population by Race and Age, Selected Mental Health Facilities, United States, 1975

SOURCE: M. J. Rosenstein and L. J. Millazzo-Sayre. **Characteristics of admissions to selected mental health facilities, 1975: An annotated book of charts and tables.** National Institute of Mental Health, 1980.

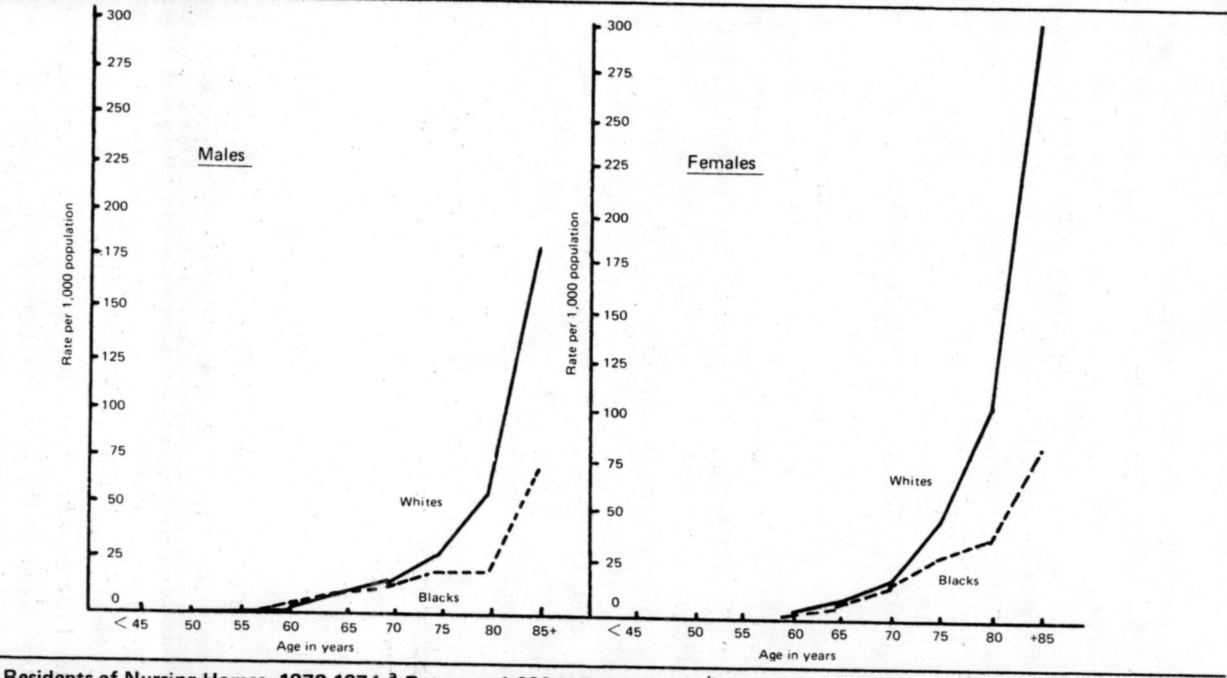

Figure 5.4 Residents of Nursing Homes, 1973-1974:[a] Rates per 1,000 U.S. Population[b] Specific for Age, Sex, and Race

a. National Center for Health Statistics. **Profile of chronic illness in nursing homes.** U.S. National Nursing Home Survey, August 1973-April 1974. Vital and Health Statistics, Series 13, No. 29, 1977.

b. Bureau of the Census. **Estimates of the population of the U.S. by age, sex, and race: 1970-1977.** Current Population Reports, Series P-25, No. 721, 1978.

these causes should be a major concern of the mental health field. In addition, the bereavement reactions related to death and the effect of the death of a family member on the role structure of the family and the resultant stresses produce high-risk populations for mental disorders.

Another important cause of death is included: lung cancer. Mortality from lung cancer is increasing rapidly among women and is still on the increase among men, for whom it is a major cause of death (Garfinkel et al., 1980). In addition, social and behavioral problems associated with lung cancer should be of interest to the mental health field. Despite increasing health risks of smoking, 42 percent of men and 32 percent of women smoke (NCHS, 1978). It is important to note that tobacco dependence is now included as a mental disorder both in ICD-9 (World Health Organization, 1977) and DSM-III (American Psychiatric Association, 1980), as rubric 305.1.

The mortality rates for each of the above causes, specific for age, sex, and race will be used to illustrate the effects of expected changes in age distribution on both total expected deaths and total (crude) death rates.

THE PROJECTIONS

Table 5.3 gives the numerical and relative increases expected in serious mental disorders, schizophrenia, senile dementia, admissions to psychiatric facilities, and residents in nursing homes.

The estimate for serious mental disorder was based on a flat 1 percent estimate. This is the group of the chronically mentally ill that has been singled out for special attention by the President's Commission (1978). It was not possible to adjust this rate for age-sex-race since the data needed to do this are not available. Persons who think this rate is too low can multiply the results given in the table for 1 percent by any factor they may desire. The important point is that whatever this rate may be, the number of such persons will increase by at least 18 percent for the white population and 39 percent for nonwhites.

For the other indexes, the increases in each racial group were based on totals that were adjusted for age and sex.[4]

Note that among the white population, the relative increases in these indexes exceed the relative increases in the total white population, with three exceptions: annual new cases of schizophrenia and point prevalence of senile dementias in the age groups 65-69 and 70-74. The reason that these conditions are increasing at a slower rate relates to the relative increase expected in the population in these age groups. With respect to schizophrenia, a decrease is expected in white persons in the age groups 15-24 years and 25-34 years, where the risk of developing this disorder is high (see Figure 5.2). For the senile dementias, the relative increase expected in the number of white persons in the age groups 65-69 and 70-74 is small, and in addition, the prevalence rates are low.

Among the black and other races group, the relative increase in numbers of cases exceeds the relative increase in their total population in every index but one: senile dementia in the age group 65-69 years. The relative increase in persons in that age group is high (35 percent); however, the prevalence rate for this age group is too low to produce a higher relative increase in number of cases.

It is important to note the differences between the relative rates of increase in the indexes shown in Table 5.3 for whites and the corresponding increases for blacks and other races. The increases in the latter group are considerably higher for every index except residents in nursing homes. Even for that index, an increase of about 42 percent would occur for the black and other races group, only slightly lower than the corresponding increase of 46 percent for whites.

The three lowest rates of increase for blacks and other races are 39 percent for annual new cases of schizophrenia, 35 percent for the 65-69-year senile dementias, 32 percent for admission to psychiatric facilities, and 42 percent for residents in nursing homes. The increases in other indexes are considerably above this. It is striking to note the expected differences between whites and other races in new cases of schizophrenia: a 5 percent increase for the former, and 39 percent for the latter. The reason for this is the expected high rate of increase in number of persons in the age groups 15-24 and 25-34 years for the black and other races group, while among whites, a decrease

Table 5.3 Effect of Population Changes in the United States, 1980-2005, on Selected Indices of Mental Disorders (assuming 1980 rates apply to the projected population for 2005)

	Number					
	White		*Black and Others*		*% Change 1980-2005*	
Index	*1980*	*2005*	*1980*	*2005*	*White*	*Black & Others*
Population	191,581,000	225,186,000	30,578,000	42,416,000	17.5	38.7
Serious Mental Disorders[a]						
(excluding senile dementia)	1,915,000	2,251,860	305,780	424,160	17.5	38.7
Schizophrenia[b]						
Annual New Cases	135,150	141,565	47,665	66,308	4.7	39.1
Cases under Care per Year	943,571	1,119,607	211,269	332,275	18.7	57.3
Senile Dementia Cases on						
a given day by Age[c]						
65-69 Years	129,369	129,637	15,383	20,754	0.2	34.9
70-74 Years	311,505	375,700	30,999	48,447	20.6	56.3
75-79 Years	443,360	647,061	37,512	69,778	45.9	86.0
80 + Years	1,016,920	1,601,475	98,963	175,917	57.5	77.7
Total 65 + Yrs.	1,901,154	2,735,873	182,857	314,896	43.9	72.2

Admissions to Psychiatric Facilities[d]	3,200,363	3,749,944	648,003	985,741	17.2	52.1
Residents in Nursing Homes[e]	1,228,769	1,800,705	67,872	96,145	46.6	41.6

a. The number of cases of serious mental disorder (excluding senile dementia) is based on an estimated worldwide prevalence rate of 1 percent for these disorders (Sartorius, 1978).

b.-e. The number of persons for each of the following indexes was obtained by applying the relevant age-specific rates for each racial group to the age distributions of the corresponding populations as estimated for 1980 and 2005 (see Table 3.1). The rates for each index, which were the most recent available, were obtained from the following references:

b. Schizophrenia: see Figure 5.2 and Babigian (1975);

c. Senile dementia: the following age-specific prevalence rates per population were used (Hagnell & Gruenberg, 1978):

Males: 65-69 yrs: 1.71; 70-74: 3.59; 75-79: 7.16; 80 + : 24.47
Females: 65-69 yrs: 1.64; 70-74: 6.14; 75-79: 13.80; 80 + : 22.50

d. Admissions to psychiatric facilities: see Figure 5.3 and National Institute of Mental Health (1981).

e. Residents in nursing homes: see Figure 5.4 and National Center for Health Statistics (1978).

is expected in the number of persons in these age groups (see Table 5.1 and Figure 5.1).

CHANGES RELATED TO MORTALITY RATES

To demonstrate the effect of the projected increase in population on the number of deaths and crude mortality rates, the mortality rates for the selected causes specific for age, sex, and cause of death for whites and the "all other" group (black and other races) were applied to the projected number of persons in each age-race group in the year 2005, specific for sex. That is, the expected number of total deaths and crude death rates were computed for race and sex and for the selected causes, assuming no change in the age-specific mortality rates during the 25-year period 1980-2005. If the age-specific death rates increase, then the expected deaths and crude death rates will increase. If the rates decrease, then the expected deaths will decrease, the amount of the decrease depending on the extent of the decrease in the age-specific rates.

Table 5.4 shows the expected changes in number of deaths for males and females, respectively, and Table 5.5 shows the corresponding changes expected in crude death rates specific for race. Inspection of Table 5.4 shows that in all but a few instances, the relative increase in deaths exceeds the relative increase in population, so that as shown in Table 5.5, the crude death rates will increase.[5]

As mentioned earlier, the number of deaths is also an indicator of the number of living persons with conditions in a population. That is, the number of deaths provides an indication of the load of morbidity and disability associated with specific conditions in a community. The latter point may be illustrated by comparing the annual number of deaths from cerebrovascular diseases in the United States in 1980 (about 216,982) with the estimated number of persons in the noninstitutional population with the condition during a year, as determined by the National Health Survey (1,656,000) (NCHS, 1974). Additional persons with these disorders are in the institutional population. For example, the number of persons in nursing homes with cerebrovascular diseases is at least 122,000 and in mental hospitals about 30,000. Thus, the total number of cases of cerebrovascular disease in the United States would be in excess of 1,800,000, and the ratio of annual cases to deaths would be more than 8 to 1.

The increases expected for deaths from homicides, suicides, automobile accidents, and all other accidents are of particular interest. These data, as we know, are only the tip of the iceberg; that is, they represent only a small fraction of the number of persons who are injured, maimed, disabled, victimized, and terrorized by events related to these external causes of morbidity, disability, and death. In addition, the number of surviving members of the victim's families and friends who are distressed, bereaved, and frightened by such events is considerable.

DISCUSSION

This chapter demonstrates the changes expected between 1981 and 2005 in the number of persons in various age groups of the population of the United States by sex and race, and illustrates the effect these changes will have on the prevalence of mental disorders, on associated chronic diseases and disabling conditions, and on the patient load of mental health services and nursing homes. These projections provide a useful basis for indicating the direction of changes likely to occur and their potential dimensions. Nevertheless, such data are still quite limited because of the lack of systematic epidemiological data on specific mental disorders in the United States. Indeed, more specific data are needed on the incidence, duration, and prevalence of specific mental disorders in various demographic groups, particularly those who are at high risk for these disorders (Hollingshead & Redlich, 1958; Bachrach, 1975; Dohrenwend et al., 1980; Gruenberg, 1981) and who are high utilizers of mental health services (Kramer et al., 1972; Kramer, 1977; NIMH, 1981a, 1981b; Gruenberg, 1980). Such rates are important because the number of persons in high-risk groups such as the following is sizable: the unmarried, never-married, separated, divorced, and widowed (Glick, 1977; U.S. Bureau of the Census, 1978b); specific ethnic groups, such as blacks, Hispanics, Native Americans, and Asians (U.S. Bureau of the

Table 5.4 Effect of Projected Population Changes in the U.S., 1980-2005[a] on the Number of Deaths from Selected Causes,[b] Specific for Race and Sex

Population and Cause of Death	*White*			*Black and Other*		
	1980	*2005*	*Percentage Change*	*1980*	*2005*	*Percentage Change*
Males						
Population (000's)	93,621	109,926	17.4	14,600	20,110	37.7
Actual Number of Deaths from:						
Cerebrov. Dis.	79,769	112,426	40.9	12,295	20,272	64.8
Cirrhosis	18,411	25,451	38.2	3,779	6,523	72.6
All accidents	64,729	76,181	17.7	12,246	18,328	49.7
Motor vehicle	30,614	34,094	11.4	5,069	7,297	44.0
All other accidents	34,115	42,087	23.4	7,177	10,831	50.9
Suicide	19,540	24,034	23.0	1,655	2,396	44.8
Homicide	8,848	10,341	16.9	8,626	14,119	63.7
Lung Cancer	63,841	84,882	33.0	8,396	14,021	67.0

FEMALES

Population(000's)	97,957	115,260	17.7	15,978	22,306	39.6
Actual Number of Deaths from:						
Cerebrov. Dis.	110,644	170,560	54.2	14,274	25,125	76.0
Cirrhosis	9,343	12,704	35.9	2,168	3,796	75.1
All accidents	27,501	36,247	31.8	4,428	6,748	52.4
Motor vehicle	10,252	11,830	15.4	1,598	2,300	43.9
All other accidents	17,249	24,417	41.6	2,830	4,448	57.2
Suicide	7,421	9,352	26.0	546	804	47.3
Homicide	2,912	3,399	16.7	2,706	3,271	20.9
Lung Cancer	19,060	25,661	34.6	2,064	3,643	76.5

SOURCES:

a. Bureau of the Census (1977)

b. National Center for Health Statistics, 1975. Cause of death is that listed in the Manual of the International Classification of Diseases (1965) A List: cerebrovascular disease, A 85; cirrhosis of liver, A102; motor vehicle accidents, AE138; all other accidents, A139-AE146; suicide and self-inflicted injury, AE147; homicide and injury purposely inflicted by other persons; legal intervention, AE148; lung cancer, A51. Deaths for 1980 and 2005 were computed by applying the reported age-specific death rates for each cause for 1975 to the projected population for the years 1980 and 2005.

Table 5.5 Projected Changes in Crude Death Rates per 100,000 Population,[a] 1980-2005, for Selected Causes in the United States by Sex and Race

Cause of Death	*Whites*			*Black and Other Races*		
	1980	*2005*	*% Change*	*1980*	*2005*	*% Change*
			Males			
Cerebrov. Dis.	85.2	102.2	20.0	84.2	100.8	19.7
Cirrhosis	19.7	23.1	17.3	25.9	32.4	25.1
All Accidents	69.1	69.3	.3	83.9	91.1	8.5
Motor Vehicle	32.7	31.0	-5.2	34.7	36.3	4.6
All other	36.4	38.3	5.2	49.2	53.9	9.6
Suicide	20.9	21.9	4.8	11.3	11.9	5.3
Homicide	9.5	9.4	-1.1	59.1	70.2	18.8
Lung Cancer	68.2	77.2	13.2	57.5	69.7	21.2
			Females			
Cerebrov. Dis.	112.9	147.9	31.0	89.3	112.6	26.1
Cirrhosis	9.5	11.0	15.8	13.6	17.0	25.0
All Accidents	30.1	31.5	4.7	27.7	30.2	9.0
Motor Vehicle	10.5	10.3	-1.9	10.0	10.3	306
All other	17.6	21.2	20.5	17.7	19.9	12.4
Suicide	7.6	8.1	6.6	3.4	3.6	5.9
Homicide	3.0	3.0	0	16.9	14.7	-13.1
Lung Cancer	19.5	22.3	14.4	12.9	16.3	26.4

a. Crude death rate for each selected cause in the years 1980 and 2005 is the ratio of the expected deaths (as shown in Table 5.4) from that cause per 100,000 population as projected for that year by the Bureau of the Census.

Census, 1978a, 1979b, 1981a, 1981b); persons living in certain types of households, such as persons living alone, female heads of households, and children living in such households (U.S. Bureau of the Census, 1978b); persons of low socioeconomic status (U.S. Bureau of the Census, 1977b, 1979a, 1979b); families with incomes at or below the poverty level and children living in such households (U.S. Bureau of the Census, 1977b); and persons of low educational attainment (U.S. Bureau of the Census, 1974).

It is to be hoped that the intensive efforts now being made by the National Institute of Mental Health (Eaton et al., 1981), the World Health Organization (1980), and others to acquire such data will fill in major gaps in our knowledge of the epidemiology of mental disorders and provide the data required to make more precise predictions of the number of cases of specific disorders, not only by age, sex, and broad racial groups used in this chapter, but by the other demographic characteristics mentioned above. Such data are needed to guide the planning and evaluation of efforts to reduce the prevalence of mental disorders and of other efforts to provide services to meet the needs of persons with such disorders.

Although there are many shortcomings and gaps in currently available morbidity and mortality statistics, this chapter demonstrates that the available statistics are sufficient to illustrate the extraordinary increases that can be expected in the number of persons who will be affected by mental disorders and by other diseases and disabling conditions that are of concern to the mental health field. This includes persons in every age group, from the youngest to the oldest. Trends similar to those in the United States are occurring worldwide. This global increase in the prevalence of chronic disease may best be characterized as a rising chronic disease pandemic (Kramer, 1980). Prevalence rates of mental disorders, Down's Syndrome, hypertensive disease, cerebrovascular disease, cirrhosis of the liver, diabetes, blindness, and other chronic conditions are increasing throughout the world.

I wish to emphasize once more the two interacting forces that are responsible for this situation. One is the large relative increase occurring in the number of persons in age groups at high risk for developing these conditions. This increases crude prevalence rates. The other mechanism is the increase in average duration of chronic diseases resulting from the successful application of techniques for arresting their fatal complications and prolonging the lives of affected individuals. This raises the age-specific prevalence rates. In the absence of effective techniques for reducing incidence, the prevalence of such diseases will continue to increase.

In the past, the public health importance of specific diseases was gauged by mortality rates. Their importance must now be gauged by prevalence rates and the extent to which they are contributing to this rising chronic-disease pandemic. Emphasis must be placed on discovering the preventable causes of the conditions that are increasing in prevalence.

Some may think that I am overly pessimistic about the future, since the underlying phenomena generating these problems are complex and complicated. On the contrary, I am optimistic about our ability to deal with these problems effectively, but it will take all of the skill, ingenuity, perseverance, and resources we can muster to do this. I have developed these data with the hope that they will promote rather than hinder our efforts to reduce the prevalence of mental disorders. To quote Frost (1936):

> Epidemiology at any given time is something more than the total of its established facts. It includes their orderly arrangement into chains of inference which extend more or less beyond the bounds of direct observation. Such of these chains as are well and truly laid guide investigation to the facts of the future; those that are ill made fetter progress.

It is my hope that the data herein presented will guide investigations not only into the facts of the future but also into our future activities. It is essential that available knowledge be applied more effectively than ever before in our efforts to reduce the prevalence of mental disorders, disorders that cause so much disability and hardship to patients, their families, significant others, and community. In addition, it is essential that new knowledge be developed to solve problems that have defied solution up to now.

The trends reported here have major implications for the training and recruitment of personnel for basic, clinical, and epidemiological research on mental disorders and associated chronic diseases; for planning and delivering mental health and associated human services; and for the financing of all such activities. As public mental health professionals, we must take such actions as may be needed to accomplish the following:

(1) increase the awareness of planners and policymakers to the seriousness of the rising pandemic of mental disorders and chronic diseases among persons of all ages and its implications for mental health, health, and related human services;
(2) develop short-, medium-, and long-range plans for developing programs for services, facilities, and manpower to deal with the problems that are certain to arise as a result of the increasing prevalence of these conditions; and
(3) develop the relevant demographic, natality, morbidity, health services, and social statistics required to plan, monitor, and evaluate the various programs.

In addition, it is essential that members of the APHA, particularly of the Mental Health Section, join forces with the members of other professional and lay organizations interested in improving the mental health of the nation. Each member of these organizations must write to our representatives in Congress and those in state legislatures emphasizing the importance of providing adequate long-term financial support for essential research activities. Of particular importance are epidemiological research—to fill in gaps in knowledge about the distribution of specific mental disorders in our population and the risk factors associated with them—and other research to discover the preventable causes of the conditions increasing in prevalence.

As members of the American Public Health Association, it is important for us to keep in mind what public health is and the goals of public health activities. These have been stated clearly by the Milbank Memorial Fund Commission on Higher Education for Public Health (1976):

> Public health is the effort organized by society to protect, promote, and restore the people's health. The programs, services, and institu-

> tions involved emphasize the prevention of disease and the health needs of the population as a whole. Public health activities change with changing technology and social values, but the goals remain the same: to reduce the amount of disease, premature death, and disease-produced discomfort and disability.

By applying this definition to our public health efforts in the mental health field, we can state the goals of our efforts as follows: to reduce the amount of mental disorders, premature death associated with these disorders, and the discomfort and disability produced by them. It is my hope that the data presented here have underscored the urgency of our developing, promoting, and obtaining support for activities to achieve these goals.

Notes

1. The two categories of race used in this chapter are (1) white and (2) black and other races. The reason for this is that the morbidity and mortality rates used were usually tabulated specific for these two categories. For the population projections used, as of 1980, blacks accounted for 85 percent of the category "black and other races." As of 2000, the corresponding proportion is estimated to be 79 percent. A goal to be achieved in the coming years is to have morbidity statistics on the mental disorders specific for the separate racial categories, as well as for the population of Spanish origin, which is the most rapidly growing of our minority populations.
2. The numbers in parentheses refer to list A of ICD-8: list of 150 causes for tabulation of morbidity and mortality.
3. The age-sex-race-specific mortality rates for these causes of death are available from the author.
4. The computations that were used in arriving at the totals given in Table 5.2 may be obtained from the author.
5. The computations that were used in arriving at the total number of deaths by cause given in Table 5.3 may be obtained from the author.

References

American Psychiatric Association. *Diagnostic and statistical manual of mental disorders* (3rd ed.) Washington, DC: Author, 1980.

BABIGIAN, H. M. Schizophrenia: Epidemiology. In A. M. Freedman et al. (Eds.), *Comprehensive textbook of psychiatry,* Vol. II. Baltimore, MD: Williams & Wilkins, 1975.

BACHRACH, L. L. *Marital status and mental disorders: An analytical review.* DHEW Publication No. (ADM)75-217. Washington, DC: Government Printing Office, 1975.

CARRUTHERS, J., EVANS, J. H., KINSLER, J., & WILLIAMS, P. Circards–A new information service on circuit design. *Wireless World,* 1972, October, 469-471.

DOHRENWEND, B. P., DOHRENWEND, B. S., GOULD, M. S., LINK, B., NEUGEBAUER, R., & WUNSCH-ITITZIG, R. *Mental illness in the United States: Epidemiological estimates.* New York: Praeger, 1980.

EATON, W. W., REGIER, D. A., LOCKE, B. Z., & TAUBE, C. A. The epidemiological catchment area program of the National Institute of Mental Health. *Public Health Reports,* 1981, *96*(4), 319-325.

FROST, W. H. Introduction. In *Snow on Cholera.* New York: The Commonwealth Fund, 1936.

GARFINKEL, L., POINDEXTER, C. E., SILVERBERG, E. Cancer statistics, 1980. *Cancer Journal for Clinicians,* 1980, *30*(1).

GLICK, P. C., & NORTON, A. J. Marrying, divorcing, and living together in the U.S. today. *Population Bulletin,* 1977, *32*(5).

GREGG, A. *The furtherance of medical research.* New Haven, CT: Yale University Press, 1941.

GRUENBERG, E. M. Failures of success. Health and Society, *The Milbank Memorial Fund Quarterly,* 1977, *4.*

GRUENBERG, E. M. Mental disorders. In J. M. Last (Ed.), *Public health and preventive medicine* (11th ed.) New York: Appleton-Century-Crofts, 1980.

GRUENBERG, E. M. Risk factor research methods. In D. A. Regier and G. Allen (Eds.), *Risk factor research in the major mental disorders.* DHHS Publication No. (ADM)81-1068. Washington, DC: Government Printing Office, 1981.

HAGNELL, O., & GRUENBERG, E. M. Personal communication, 1978.

HOLLINGSHEAD, A. B., & REDLICH, F. C. *Social class and mental illness.* New York: John Wiley, 1958.

KRAMER, M. Population changes and schizophrenia, 1970-1985. In L. C. Wynne (Ed.), *The nature of schizophrenia.* New York: John Wiley, Inc., 1975.

KRAMER, M. *Psychiatric services and the changing institutional scene, 1950-1985.* DHEW Publication No. (ADM)77-433. Washington, DC: Government Printing Office, 1977.

KRAMER, M. The rising pandemic of mental disorders and associated chronic diseases and disabilities. *Acta psychiat scand,* 1980, *285*(62).

KRAMER, M., POLLACK, E. S., REDICK, R. W., & LOCKE, B. Z. *Mental disorders/ suicide.* Cambridge, MA: Harvard University Press, 1972.

Milbank Memorial Fund Commission. *Higher education for public health.* New York: Produst, 1976.

National Center for Health Statistics. *Prevalence of chronic circulatory conditions, U.S., 1972.* Washington, DC: Government Printing Office, 1974.

National Center for Health Statistics. *Profile of chronic illness in nursing homes.* Washington, DC: Government Printing Office, 1977.

National Center for Health Statistics. *Health, United States, 1978.* DHEW Publication No. (PHS)78-1232. Washington, DC: Government Printing Office, 1978.

National Center for Health Statistics. *Vital Statistics of the United States, 1975.* Washington, DC: Government Printing Office, 1979.

National Center for Health Statistics. *Vital Statistics of the United States, 1977: Lifetables.* Hyattsville, MD: Author, 1980.

National Institute of Mental Health. *Characteristics of admissions to selected mental health facilities, 1975.* NHHS Publication No. (ADM)81-1005, Washington, DC: Government Printing Office, 1981. (a)

National Institute of Mental Health. *Hispanic Americans and mental health services.* DHHS Publication No. (ADM)80-1006. Washington, DC: Government Printing Office, 1981. (b)

The President's Commission on Mental Health. *Report to the President.* Washington, DC: Government Printing Office, 1978.

REGIER, D. A., GOLDBERG, I. D., & TAUBE, C. A. The de facto U.S. mental health services system. *Archives of General Psychiatry,* 1978, *35,* 685-693.

SARTORIUS, N. Personal communication, 1978.

U.S. Bureau of the Census. *Population of the United States, trends and prospects: 1950-1990.* Current Population Reports, Series P-23, No. 49. Washington, DC: Government Printing Office, 1974.

U.S. Bureau of the Census. *Projections of the population of the United States: 1977-2005.* Current Population Reports, Series P-25, No. 704. Washington, DC: Government Printing Office, 1977. (a)

U.S. Bureau of the Census. *Chracteristics of the population below the poverty level: 1975.* Current Population Reports, Series P-60, No. 106. Washington, DC: Government Printing Office, 1977. (b)

U.S. Bureau of the Census. *Social and economic characteristics of the metropolitan and nonmetropolitan population, 1977 and 1970.* Current Population Report, Series P-23, No. 75. Washington, DC: Government Printing Office, 1978. (a)

U.S. Bureau of the Census. *Marital status and living arrangements.* Current Population Reports, Series P-20, No. 338. Washington, DC: Government Printing Office, 1978. (b)

U.S. Bureau of the Census. *Social and economic characteristics of the older population: 1978.* Current Population Reports, Series P-23, No. 85. Washington, DC: Government Printing Office, 1979. (a)

U.S. Bureau of the Census. *Persons of Spanish origin in the United States: March, 1978.* Current Population Reports, Series P-20, No. 339. Washington, DC: Government Printing Office, 1979. (b)

U.S. Bureau of the Census. *Median age data, other 1980 census results released.* Washington, DC: Author, 1981. (a)

U.S. Bureau of the Census. *Age, sex, race and Spanish origin of the population by regions, divisions and states, 1980.* Washington, DC: Government Printing Office, 1981. (b)

U.S. Department of Labor. *Employment and training report of the president, 1979.* Washington, DC: Government Printing Office, 1979.

U.S. Department of Labor. *Recent trends in the labor force and participation rates, 1980.* Washington, DC: Government Printing Office, 1980.

World Health Organization. *International classification of diseases: Manual of the international statistical classification of diseases, injuries and causes of death.* Geneva, 1977.

World Health Organization. *Sixth report on the world health situation, 1973-1977,* Part I: *Global Analysis.* Geneva, 1980.

Chapter 6

EPIDEMIOLOGY AND MENTAL HEALTH POLICY

NORMAN SARTORIUS

The fact that there are some 300 million people in the world who have mental disorders of sufficient severity to mar their lives (Sartorius, 1978) should cause an influx of funds for facilities providing treatment and searching for better ways of handling mental disorders.

The fact that it is highly probable that we are facing a pandemic of disability (see Kramer, Chapter 5, this volume), and that very frequently the difference between compensated functional limitation and severe disability lies in the attitudes of the impaired and those who surround them, should make psychosocial factors a central target for the research and action of those concerned with disability prevention and rehabilitation.

The fact that the world is undergoing rapid socioeconomic and cultural changes and that such changes are likely to increase in rate and magnitude over the next ten to twenty years should lead to an increased emphasis on the mental health effects of such changes on individuals, their families, and communities expressed both in declarations and in allocations of funds for action and research to prevent untoward side-effects and to optimize development.

Yet none of this is happening on anything like a worldwide, significant scale. In spite of evidence that epidemiological (and other) research has produced, the mental health sciences have low priority, and mental health policy seems to be made without much regard for data about mental disorder or for facts about the promotion of mental health. The care of the mentally ill is given low priority and their needs are now neglected. Behavioral science gets little money for research and even less recognition, and major sociocultural and economic interventions and policy changes are carried out without seeking or heeding advice from mental health specialists.

This appears to be so regardless of whether the debate concerns the global, regional, or national situation. The epidemiology of mental disorders seems to have produced results that no one but other epidemiologists and birds of the same scientific feather want to see.

WHO LISTENS TO EPIDEMIOLOGISTS?

The health decision makers apparently do not listen to what scientists say. They act, paying no attention to findings of painstaking research; they commit avoidable errors without reasonable justification; rather than using data, they fund more research of the same kind applied for by researchers who are given ample proof that none will listen to what they have to say once their investigation is done.

According to all accounts, those outside the health sector—as well as the general public—are no different. Although epidemiological information about mental disease, impairment, and disability is offered to all, most people pay no serious attention to it; they tend to give preference to data about sources of pleasure and ways of increasing their physical and mental capacity. Doctors and other professionals who are in the business of healing don't seem to care too much either. They state with much conviction that they have rarely had a clear demonstration that knowing an epidemiological fact had a direct practical consequence and was useful for their daily work.

Thus, it is said, neither decision makers in health nor those who make policy in other social sectors, nor the general public, nor the professional groups listen to epidemiologists. They act for a variety of emotional reasons, disregarding evidence that epidemiologists produce. They seem to prefer irrationality in decision making and do not seem to be the worse for it.

If that is so, then the famous dicta about the utility of epidemiological research for the variety of purposes that Morris (1978) and so many others have so eloquently described are invalid, and it is only the epidemiologists who are foolish enough to believe that their data matter in policy making.

On the other hand, it is true that it is impossible to exclude the possibility that on some occasions, in some countries, and for a variety of unrelated reasons, epidemiological data did in fact have direct influence on decision making and policy formulation. The recent examination of the epidemiological evidence by the President's Commission on Mental Health (1978), the fact that the decision about the changes in policy concerning old age homes in Denmark was taken using results of Strömgren's investigations (Hafner, 1979), and the reduction of the number of hospital beds in the UK (Tooth and Brooke, 1961) were among a considerable number of events that were suggested to me as examples of the impact that data have had on policy formulation. But for each example of their impact, there were many of the lack of any effect. Furthermore, it proved to be very difficult to produce any examples of the impact of data on policy in most countries. Also, on close examination, some of the examples of impact seem to be able to withstand only very superficial scrutiny and quickly dissolve when seriously studied. It thus appears that there are many who seem to share the conviction that epidemiological and other data have little, if any, influence on mental health policy, action, or evaluation, and that the situation is in fact getting worse—that is, that more and more data are produced and that they have less and less impact.

Since no one has yet produced definite evidence of our ability to measure the impact of epidemiological information, I feel that I am allowed to speculate and overgeneralize about the apparent lack of influence that epidemiological data have on mental health policy making and offer some hypotheses to explain this troublesome state of affairs.

I would like to propose four hypotheses to explain the situation: My first hypothesis is that the lamentation about the lack of readiness to use epidemiological data is unfounded and exaggerated, and that it stems from producers of irrelevant data that they present in an incomprehensible manner to the wrong people.

My second hypothesis is that the lamentation is well justified, and that nobody in policy-making circles wants epidemiological evidence until after decisions are made—when data will be requested to support those decisions.

My third hypothesis is that the data which are produced do in fact get used, but that between the time of production and the time of use there is an incubation (latency) period during which decisions based on data of an earlier vintage are taken. Data in this hypothesis have a modus operandi like slow viruses; once produced and ingested, they will have an effect, but later—much later. In between either nothing happens or effects of an even earlier data input are felt.

Finally, there is a fourth hypothesis, by which it is assumed that all three of the others are to some extent true.

The first hypothesis—about the irrelevance of data produced by the epidemiology of mental disorders—is built on the fact that for a variety of reasons inherent in research and policy making, it is only extremely rarely possible to produce data that are relevant for the policy options available to decision makers at the time of data production. Valid or invalid information is relevant only when it can be directly related in time and space to the concerns and needs of the consumer—in this instance, the policy makers. Hence, even the most fascinating findings are irrelevant for policy making unless they are ready just when and where needed.

Data are also irrelevant for policy making if they are expressed in a register different from that which the policy maker uses. To state, for example, that there are 20 new cases of schizophrenia per 100,000 inhabitants per year is not relevant data for most decision makers having to allocate resources, marshal funds, protect the government from embarrassment, get reelected, and satisfy vociferous professions, pressure groups, and lobbies. The 20 per 100,000 figure should come to them with additional facts, including, for example, the likely prevalence of schizophrenia for the area for which they are responsible; figures about the level of disability that the disease is likely to cause in that culture; evidence on whether it matters that the disease is left untreated; and information on what currently happens to those ill and whether some unpleasant consequences for the community, some important subgroup of the population, the health services, and/or for the decision makers will occur if nothing is done. The swift reaction—almost an overkill—to information about drug dependence in adolescents from middle- and upper-class families that recently occurred in some Asian countries makes the point about information relevance better than any theoretical treatise, particularly when this reaction is compared to the sluggish shrugging of shoulders usually given in answer to information about, say, a 100 times higher prevalence of mental retardation in those same countries.

PRESENTATION

Presenting information in a manner incomprehensible to decision makers is another reason for a lack of reaction. "Incomprehensible" does not refer only to an intellectual understanding of the figures presented; it also refers to the connotational aspects of words about mental health problems.

Epidemiologists and other mental health specialists tend to operate on the belief that decision makers are like themselves; in fact, they usually are not. Barbara Wooton (1980) recently wrote about this phenomenon, trying to explain why judges do not do very well with some offenders. She wrote:

> Judges and magistrates seem to think that offenders' mental processes are much what they imagine their own would be in similar circumstances, and they envisage both the man in the dock and themselves as, potentially at least, liable to similar temptations. In looking into his heart, they appear in fact only to see what lurks in their own. Legislators likewise, in drafting the criminal law, seem equally disposed to draw upon introspective evidence: as when advocates of capital punishment project images of how they would refrain from carrying guns on a robbery if to do so would put their own lives at risk.
>
> Up to a point, of course, this works. . . . But the point at which the courts' traditionalist psychology really breaks down is in relation to what are often called "motiveless crimes," that is to say crimes which we cannot imagine ourselves committing or even being

> tempted to commit. To illustrate: when I used to hear shoplifting cases on a London West End bench, offenders who came from overseas seemed to fall into two classes: the first consisted of European students collecting useful articles either for themselves or for presents. They would usually have only about £5 left and were due to return home next week, so no effective penalty could be imposed. The others generally came from further away and had committed more trivial thefts, but often carried substantial sums of money. Within the horizons of our criminal justice system, the first lot are comprehensible (but intractable), the second merely incomprehensible.

The producer of data about mental disorders frequently appears to the decision maker as the motiveless criminal to Wooton's magistrate: Why, for example, should anyone want to do much about the mildly retarded? They do not seem to request it, their relatives do not complain too much, they will not die from it, and anyway, the world is made of all kinds of people. Why, in other words, do anything? But the value system of the epidemiologist who believes that the enhancement of mental capacity and a full mental life are a most desirable goal of health efforts is not necessarily the value system of other health professionals, including the decision maker—a fact which, if forgotten, will ensure that data are not comprehended in their full significance and potential impact.

Irrelevance and incomprehension of data can also be achieved by presenting material to the wrong people. Only too frequently epidemiologists forget to apply their own science to patterns of decision making in their own setting so as to ensure that their words reach the one person who matters, somewhere in the system. True, methods for the study of social bonds and operations research on decision making are not the most advanced of epidemiological techniques, but not even the rudimentary tools of that ilk are used in searching for the right person to whom data should be given.

Not infrequently, after several bitter experiences, epidemiologists will withdraw from attempts to make their data bear on policy making, concentrating instead on eremitical jeremiads written only for their epidemiologist colleagues, without any effort to give their papers the taste of life that might help to convince people who are not of their opinion.

WHAT DECISION MAKERS REACT TO

Decision makers are more likely to react to the statement that in Europe, for each traffic accident death, there is also a suicide death, and that for every person dying from suicide, there are ten who attempt it—and whose treatment costs a great deal of money—than they are to the statement that there are some 14 deaths per 100,000 inhabitants per year, mostly among the elderly and often among those with a chronic, incurable disease. It is as if, in addition to training in the preparation of scientific reports, the psychiatric epidemiologist has to have another course on presenting data for people with little time, little money, under stress, and without a built-in weakness for psychological matters.

The second hypothesis is that in fact, those who have to make decisions and formulate policies do not want to hear (or do not care) about epidemiological findings concerning mental disorders. Reasons for this may be found easily. First, many of the health decision makers in the world today were qualified without any training in mental health matters. They were perhaps exposed—for a short period of time early in their training—to a week or so of visitation to the local lunatic asylum, during which time they were greatly amused by the curious behavior of the inmates, happy that these crazies were locked up rather than roaming the streets, and mildly disgusted over the hygienic conditions of the wards. Sometimes they may have also felt genuine sympathy and pitied those kept in the institutions, but were probably reassured by their teachers that little if anything could be done to ease the lot of those inside.

Second, most decision makers and policy formulators dislike scientists for what they perceive as their lack of concern about the grueling business of administering health or other services. By and large, the general public dislike the "eggheads" as well, for this and other reasons, making it possible for the decision makers to find support for their views in popular beliefs. Proposals that come from scientists are, in the opinion and experience of decision makers, likely to be unrealistic and often difficult to explain. Also, they lack soothing information about the way to handle the difficulties that will undoubtedly arise if a decision is made, and thus one option given preference over others; nor is there in most proposals much information coming from scientists about the indirect cost of accepting them—for example, in terms of identifying what can be done to pacify groups whose proposals are rejected when another option is chosen.

Third, epidemiologists often present their data forgetting that decision makers and legislators—as all other people—have to hear the same fact frequently and from many different people before they start to believe in its veracity. A single presentation, no matter how solid the evidence, will not produce much reaction, even if comprehensible, timely, relevant, and true. The same finding must also be heard from other sources, on other occasions. Policy making is usually based on—but rarely directed by—data. Facts other than numerical accounts of disease prevalence enter into decision making with force at all levels. As a result, political interests and considerations may effectively reduce the willingness of decision makers to listen and act, be they the politics of an office, a town, a country, or a continent.

Fourth, the time scale of legislators and policy makers differs from that of epidemiologists. The latter may propose preventive measures that will have an effect in 20 years, while the decision makers' scale of reckoning does not exceed, say, two years, by which time he must have results of his policy in hand, ready to show.

Fifth, decision makers are not by nature people who like to be told what to do. They are leaders because of their personality and the belief of those whom they lead that they know what to do better than others around them. Most leaders will try to live up to this image and consequently advice, given in the manner of an academic teacher (as is the habit of many scientists), is not likely to be heeded, particularly if given publicly.

Sixth, for a long time psychiatry—compared to other disciplines, such as surgery—had no effective treatment methods in its arsenal. True, more recently there is talk about psychopharmacology, but after all, these are only symptomatic treatments (as if digitalis treatment were not), and many people do not agree with their effectiveness. Evidence about the effectiveness of psychiatric treatment is usually not common knowledge.

The decision makers therefore feel that the chances to achieve nothing are great and that action may be wasteful.

Seventh, while general epidemiology has a place of honor in public health and in health policy making, and a remarkable record of achievements to its credit, the epidemiology of mental disorders is a less well established and recognized discipline, still under a challenge to produce evidence comparable to that of general epidemiology. The epidemiologist dealing with mental disorders may therefore be less well accepted by decision makers and not infrequently distrusted by psychiatrists, who then inform the decision makers about their distrust and give them different advice.

Eighth, the psychiatrist and his professional colleagues usually don't have the image of "gung ho" managers of field campaigns or otherwise quick-moving, active "doers"—they are usually seen as contemplative types, sometimes a bit bizarre as well. They are therefore the natural opposites of decision makers in any field, including health, and unlikely to inspire confidence that funds given them will bring quick returns.

Ninth, decision makers are used to react to change, emergencies, imminent doom, or embarrassment. By nature, mental illness is neither epidemic nor news; in one form or another, it has always been present, and for a long time there was little that could be done about it. Therefore, the decision maker accepts epidemiological findings about mental disorders with quiet resignation and no impatience to act.

Finally, most decision makers see mental health problems as competing with other health problems. This is easily the most damaging fallacy of all: Physical disease does not render people immune to mental disorder. In fact, mental health aspects of overall health programs are usually of decisive importance for treatment of individuals and health promotion of communities. But to convince decision makers that rather than competing, mental and physical health efforts should be handled as complementary tasks is a difficult proposition at any time.

My third hypothesis to explain the lack of impact of information from psychiatric epidemiology on policy making is that the lack of impact is only apparent and that mental disease evidence—as any other evidence, for that matter—takes many years to seep through and activate policy-making mechanisms. This slow-virus hypothesis of information use seems to find its confirmation in many instances—for example, that of smoking. The evidence that led to whatever changes have been made in legislation, behavior, and so forth was released many years before its effects became apparent.

Similar long-term effects of information could be presupposed for a variety of data input, in health and elsewhere. It is more difficult to prove or disprove this hypothesis. Also, it is disquieting to speculate about the consequences that it would have if confirmed. First, it would be necessary to restrict data input to information that is likely to retain its relevance for at least 20 years or more. Second, there is no way in which one could disclaim responsibility for not using data in decision making, as is often done now, claiming that epidemiological information does not matter. Finally, if true in psychiatric epidemiology, this law probably holds in other fields as well, and effects of measures such as the abolition of capital punishment will be irrevocably present in, say, a generation from now.

My own preference would be to believe that all three hypotheses are in part correct. It is true that decision makers—most of the time and for a variety of reasons—are content not to have to introduce changes in health policies. It is also true that mental disease epidemiologists often produce data at the wrong time in the wrong form, and that they try to give it to the wrong people for the wrong reasons.

Finally, it cannot be excluded that the nature of public action is such that there will be a long delay between information input and policy change, regardless of subjects and individuals. This is at least a consoling thought for the many whose data seemed to make no impact after they were published or handed to authorities.

There is every reason to pursue action in three of these hypothetical areas—that is, to make an effort to change the attitudes of decision makers, to educate psychiatric epidemiologists, and to carry out research on the temporal aspects of data effects. Perhaps that will help give the data base in psychiatric epidemiology a chance to have as much practical impact as its theoretical significance deserves.

EPIDEMIOLOGY OF HEALTH

Should all this succeed—and I hope it will—still a new danger arises. Even at its best, the epidemiology of mental disorders will never be in a position to provide data on which to base action to promote mental health. For this, mental health policy makers will have to reach into philosophy, religion, ethics, and history. Decision makers may be reluctant to do so. It may be more comfortable to extrapolate from mental disorder to mental health, and from disease prevention to health promotion. This kind of thinking and action, unfortunately, already happens in a variety of ways. If only we could remove mental illness, it is said, mental health would improve. If only we knew causes of mental disorder, we could prevent it, and a blissful existence would begin. Somehow, some parts of the disease model from physical medicine are forgotten when mental disorder is debated. Lifting a boat from the ocean and putting it ashore for repainting does not change the ocean. The successful treatment of depression removes depression; it does not change mental health. It is no doubt useful and important for factors that may cause or exacerbate mental illness to be recommended as targets for public health action; however, removing these factors will not in itself promote mental health, nor may it be taken as an excuse for not doing something else about it.

Among the steps that are necessary if we want to start serious action in this field is that we shall have to promote much more seriously an epidemiology of states of health rather than only of mental disease. Systematic study of social bonds, factors promoting psychosocial development in adverse conditions, attitudes about sickness in oneself and others, the effectiveness of methods to avoid lifestyles conducive to failure, and studies of the distribution and nature of states of health and functioning are probably among the topics that such an epidemiology could study so as to be able to provide decision makers with information on what to do to enhance mental health and enable people to have a full mental life, which after all is what makes them human.

Improving our mental life is the ultimate goal of our existence. It is that portion of life which has to include coping with mental or physical diseases, worries, happiness, ideas, and perceptions. Removing mental disease is a noble goal that can facilitate a fuller mental life. In this sense, mental disorder epidemiology can make a contribution to policies leading to better health. It cannot and should not attempt to do more. For that, we have not only to develop an epidemiology of states of health, but also accept the predominant importance of mental life as a new basis for our action, for all other health action, and indeed for all social endeavor.

References

HAFNER, H. Estimation of needs on the basis of field survey findings. *Estimating needs for mental health care.* Geneva: World Health Organization, 1979.

MORRIS, J. N. *The uses of epidemiology.* New York: Churchill, 1978.

President's Commission on Mental Health. *Report to the President.* Washington, DC: Goverment Printing Office, 1978.

SARTORIUS, N. The new mental health programs of WHO. *Interdisciplinary Science Review,* 1978, *3,* 202-206.

TOOTH, G. C. and BROOKE, E. M. Trends in the mental hospital population and their effect on future planning. *Lancet,* 1961, *1,* 710-713.

WOOTON, B. Psychiatry, ethics and the criminal law. *British Journal of Psychiatry,* 1980, *136,* 525-532.

Part III

ISSUES IN MANPOWER AND TRAINING

Chapter 7

TRENDS IN TRAINING AND PRACTICE

NOLAN E. PENN

Twenty-five years ago, during the middle 1950s, our nation was simultaneously attempting to recover from its involvement in the Korean conflict while in the midst of rapidly advancing technology. We first observed the launching of Russia's satellite, Sputnik, and then of our own space satellites, later capping these experiences by placing American citizens on the surface of the moon. Equally remarkable during this period, I believe, were some of the new and significant discoveries in the mental health field. A number of these important events will be discussed here, and my chapter will attend to trends in training and manpower during the past 25 years.

During World War II we discovered the extended benefits of behavioral therapies and psychodynamic interventions for disorders other than the well-known major classifications, such as combat neuroses. These successes gave us the rationale for obtaining governmental support to expand VA neuropsychiatric services and to gain support for professional training in the four core mental health disciplines: psychiatry, psychology, social work, and nursing.

New therapies and treatment programs were developed in the 1950s, coinciding with an increase in personnel in the state hospital system, increases in hospital admissions, and the utilization of developing child guidance and outpatient clinics.

Until the late 1950s, the principal mode of care for severely disturbed psychiatric patients was long-term hospitalization. The 1950s and 1960s produced two monumental achievements: psychoactive medications in the 1950s, and the Community Mental Health Centers Act in 1963. The first of these started the deinstitutionalization of a great number of "chronic patients," and the second provided for a "care in the community" program and concept.

A new kind of mental health worker was created in the 1960s called the "paraprofessional"; in fact, there were a number of terms applied, all meaning "something less than." As a group, in a variety of settings, they did more than some of the core professions in providing direct care for the mentally disturbed. Paraprofessional groups were created when we were warned by the final report of the Joint Commission on Mental Illness and Health (1961) that the number of core professionals would never be sufficient to deal with the care of those in need.

EXTENDING MENTAL HEALTH SERVICES

The legislation in 1963 (President's Commission, 1978b), which established the Community Mental Health Centers program and which moved us from dependency on the custodial-oriented state hospital to community-based care, also gave entitlement to care to every citizen, an idea that grew out of the civil rights movement and the legislation of the 1950s and 1960s. This idea of citizen rights permeates many areas, including consumer rights, minority rights, employee rights, rights of the handicapped, the aged, and of women, children, and students. The affirmation of individual rights of all U.S. citizens to mental health care that is available, accessible, acceptable, and affordable has been the basis for the expansion of both private and public services, but more importantly, it was the basis for assuring the availability of mental health service delivery personnel for persons lacking such care: the rural, the poor, minorities, the aged, the chronically mentally ill, the mentally retarded, alcoholics, and drug abusers.

Some trends occurring during the past 15-25 years were reported by the President's Commission on Mental Health (1978: 423-426). Some had implications for mental health personnel that are being articulated in recent judicial decrees related to patients' rights. For example, the right to treatment, the right to treatment in the least restrictive setting (at home in the community), the right of informed consent to treatment procedures, and the right to refuse treatment. Other trends that affected the overall human services, as well as the mental health field, were: deinstitutionalization and the development of community-based services; the development of self-help groups and renewed interest in natural systems of support in neighborhoods and communities (e.g., churches, friends, lodges); greater interdependence of these systems as they all work with multiproblem persons and families in the communities; sharing of not only the same kinds of personnel, but even of the same persons over a period of time; innovative service delivery programs; preventive activities and the promotion of well-being, in addition to remedial and supportive services; comprehensive state and local planning programs, including planning for personnel; and the trends to demand accountability in terms of cost control, productivity, and quality assurance.

The foregoing trends have affected personnel in the mental health field, including hiring, training, deployment, relocation, and retention. In addition, there have been some specific trends in the mental health field itself that have affected personnel needs. They are: new techniques of intervention; the movement of all types of mental health professionals into positions of top administrative leadership in mental health programs; the trend to provide for the rehabilitation and restoration of patients to community settings, rather than simple diagnosis and treatment; the trend for persons suffering from a wider variety of mental and emotional problems to seek treatment from mental health programs; and the trend of society to define problems as mental health problems that were formerly criminal justice problems; and of late, the trend to redefine or remove from the psychiatric "disordered" classification behaviors that may be viewed as harmless social deviancies.

OUTPATIENT SERVICES

Let us turn briefly to a review of some of the workforce figures in the mental health system over the past 25 years. Prior to 1955, the state hospital was the dominant care institution in the mental health system. In 1955, with the introduction of psychoactive drugs, we saw a continuing decline in the state hospital census over the next 20 years—changing from about 750,000 in 1955 to about 200,000 in 1975, and the census continues to drop. In 1975, over 6.5 million people were treated in the specialized mental health sector, both public and private. Many were seen in more than a single location. About 25 percent were seen in inpatient units; however, less than 10 percent of these were in state and country hospitals. Most persons needing this type of service were being seen in general and VA hospitals, or in CMHC-affiliated units (President's Commission, 1978b: 426).

In addition to those seen in specialized units, about 1.3 million persons were seen in the private practice sector, using the services of psychiatrists and psychologists, primarily. Nearly 150,000 students sought help from campus clinics. It is believed that this total of 6.7 million people seen in specialized units accounts for about 21 percent (8 million) of the estimated 32 million believed to suffer some emotional disorder that could be assisted by the mental health system. The bulk of this remaining group were treated in hospitals without separate psychiatric units, and at least 207,000 were cared for in nursing homes. About 19 million (60 percent) of the total 32 million were treated as outpatients by nonpsychiatrically trained physicians and in medical clinics or hospital emergency rooms. Finally, nearly 7 million people were estimated to have received no services or to have sought advice from the social services sector or from community support systems, such as churches and self-help groups (President's Commission, 1978b: 427). As one might suspect, even in 1980 there are no data to describe the effectiveness of the services provided or of the skills of general health care or social service practitioners in diagnosing and treating mental disorder. Some evidence suggests that many of the most severely disturbed people are currently seen in specialized facilities by mental health professionals in private practice.

In summary, since 1955 we have experienced a substantial increase in the use of outpatient services; twelvefold more than in 1955. The rate and number of inpatient treatment episodes have continued to increase, but there are fewer patients in state hospitals and more patients in general hospitals, many without psychiatric wards. The private practice sector has continued to grow rapidly in recent years, largely due to the addition of psychologists and social workers to this core group (President's Commission, 1978b: 427).

Since 1955, we have experienced a broadening of both the range of mental health facilities and the types of services provided by these facilities. Inpatient, outpatient, transitional, and indirect services have increased the range of services, while client assessments, physical and psychological therapies, educational and rehabilitation services, social and supportive services, indirect community services, and administrative and managerial services all contributed to extensions of the types of services. While the latter refer to activities directed at maintaining and improving the mental health system, rather than to clients or communities, these are deemed to be important to personnel changes (President's Commission, 1978b: 427).

STAFFING PATTERNS

How have staffing patterns changed during the past 25 years? Psychiatrists, psychologists, social workers, and psychiatric nurses provided most of the mental health services up until 1955. Since then, substantial changes have occurred within each of these disciplines, and additional types of providers have entered the care delivery field—for example, baccalaureate and master's-level health professionals, and A.A. degree mental health workers (President's Commission, 1978b: 431).

From 1972 to 1976, the number of full-time positions in the mental health field increased by 13 percent. Psychologists, social workers, "other mental health professionals," and psychiatric nurses experienced the largest relative increases between

1974 and 1976: 21 percent, 17 percent, and 16 percent, respectively. The less-than-B.A. degree categories increased slightly. Three disciplines experienced decreases between 1974 and 1976: L.P.N.s and L.V.N.s showed an 11 percent decrease, physical health professionals and assistants had an 8 percent decrease, and nonpsychiatric physicians experienced a 5 percent decline. The net effects of these changes was an increased proportion of professionals as total staff for patient care for each of the three years (1974-1976): 27 percent, 32 percent, and 24 percent, respectively. Government data reveal shifting staffing patterns in the past two to five years. State mental hospitals (mostly providing inpatient services) are primarily staffed by paraprofessionals—aides and attendants—however, the percentage of professional patient care staff is rising. The CMHCs (providing outpatient care mostly) are staffed primarily by professionals, and the percentage of paraprofessionals is dropping. Slightly more than 50 percent of the full-time patient care staff is from the four major professional disciplines—however, the percentage of psychologists and social workers has been rising, while the proportion of psychiatrists and nurses has been falling (President's Commission, 1978b: 431; Bass, 1978; Rosenstein & Taube, 1978; Taube, 1974, 1976; NIMH, 1970).

The professional workforce has grown rapidly in recent decades. There were 7,100 psychiatrists in 1950 and 28,000 in 1980. Recently, the American Psychiatric Association predicted the need for 50,000 psychiatrists in 1980 (Hausman, 1980). There were 7,300 psychologists in 1950 and nearly 50,000 in 1980. Both groups are mostly white, practice in large, urban, wealthy sections of the United States, study and know very little about children, families, the elderly, the poor, and the various ethnic and cultural groups in the United States. This statement is especially true for psychiatry. These professionals are employed mainly in CMHCs and private practice, not usually in hospitals. There were 20,000 to 100,000 social workers in 1955 and about 300,000 today, depending on how one makes the estimate. While this group has more women and minorities, they do not necessarily know more about them than the other professions. These figures contain all categories of social work service and do not refer only to the master's degree.

Today, there are about 1 million nurses, about 30,000 of whom are psychiatric nurses, but only a few are fully trained at the master's degree level (President's Commission, 1978b: 432-439). Due to the nature of the resource data on nurses, there seems to be some uncertainty about these figures; they are considered in some nursing quarters to be an overestimate of the number of completely trained registered nurses.

SUPPLY AND DISTRIBUTION

Issues related to the supply and distribution of personnel can be summarized briefly as follows: More personnel, in general, are needed to perform all types of activities needed in the mental health system—help in housing, employment, income maintenance, vocational training, and the like—these services are to be administered (and we know that people seek them when coming to the mental health system for help). Geographic maldistribution continues to be a real problem. New medical school graduates, we are told, are not enchanted by psychiatry, and we need a continuous influx of nurses, from the R.N. diploma level through to the master's degree level.

But education requires commitment to lengthy periods of study, and almost all students require some stipend support in today's inflationary and recessive economy. In addition, the incoming supply of foreign trained physicians, upon which the mental health system had developed a dependency relationship, will be drastically reduced as a result of the recent Health Professions and Educational Assistance Act of 1976. This phenomenon, combined with fewer than 1 percent of the new medical school graduates choosing psychiatry, will decrease our supply of psychiatrists to an enormous degree. Thus, if our nation believes that an adequate supply is vital to the provision of mental health services of all varieties, we must make the profession more attractive to potential new medical applicants, as does any other discipline declared to have a shortage (President's Commission, 1978b: 461-463).

This same report (p. 456) informs us that distribution is a critical problem as the core professionals continue to congregate in the major cities of the wealthier states. It has been estimated that 68 percent of all counties in the United States have no psychiatrists–most of these are rural, although some are within driving distance of a city. But due to the expense involved, this latter aspect does not help the poor to obtain psychological counseling. Some states have a ratio of one psychiatrist per 25,000 population, while other states have one psychiatrist for each 5,000 population. About 82 percent of all psychiatrists practice in cities of 100,000 or greater. Rural areas, unable to provide the many attractions and amenities wished for, fail to attract qualified professionals from the four core professions.

Our training institutions fail in two ways to help this situation: one, they do not admit and graduate sufficient numbers of the type of qualified professionals who might work in the less wealthy urban centers and in the rural areas where the poor and the ethnic minorities reside; and two, the curricula of most university medical and professional schools contain very little to nothing about the culture, issues, and special problems of the poor, ethnic minorities, the aged, families, and children. The training of professionals must include content on the foregoing groups, as well as collaborative work situations with ethnic minority patients, professionals, and "other mental health workers", both professional and paraprofessional. In the meantime, while the mental health system continues to consist of a white majority, whites must be sensitized through training to the needs of other cultures. Perhaps then more ethnic minorities will come for care and not drop out after a single visit or two. The content of such recommended training could be taught by faculty from these ethnic minority groups. For example, learning from native healers from the many subcultures in the United States could be crucial to the development of a better and more interactive mental health delivery system.

ETHNIC AND RACIAL MINORITIES

The problem with admitting ethnic and racial minorities to mental health training programs continues to be most critical. Fewer than 2 percent of all fully trained psychiatrists are Black. Complete data on the other ethnic groups are difficult to interpret, but we remain concerned over their low numbers.

Ph.D.-level psychologists are represented at less than 1 percent in each of the major ethnic groups: Black, Hispanic, Asian-American, and Native American. Social work and nursing have more minorities, but still the numbers trained at the highest professional levels, B.S.W. and M.S.W., are embarrassingly too few. Numbers of trainees from the various ethnic groups are also low: 3.4 percent of psychiatry trainees are Black; 6 percent of the Ph.D.s awarded in 1976 were to members of ethnic minorities, as were 23 percent of the bachelor of social work degrees and 17 percent of the master's degrees in social work; and 18 percent of the R.N.s graduating in 1975 were members of ethnic minorities (Bass, 1978: 458-459).

Any discussion about personnel must speak to the quality of and access to education. Training is costly; therefore, it must be financed. The NIMH's initial intention was to increase the number of trained mental health personnel, as well as to improve the quality of education in the field. The training budget of the NIMH was $1 million in 1948, $4.8 million in 1955, $24.8 million in 1960, and $120 million in 1969 (President's Commission, 1978b). This report notes that the major funding emphasis was on training in the four core professions, although some was given to the training of paraprofessionals and other special projects. In 1972, the NIMH supported the training of 44 percent of psychiatry residents, 28 percent of clinical psychology graduate students, 38 percent of M.S.W. students, and 90 percent of M.A. psychiatric nurse students.

Since 1972, NIMH, VA, and other training funds have been reduced drastically, particularly in psychiatry. Inadequate funding will cut back on innovations, reduce the quality of education, and make it difficult to recruit from the ethnic minority groups. In 1981, the elimination of future clinical training support at the NIMH for all mental health care professions was a policy goal of the Reagan Administration; funding is scheduled to be drastically reduced in fiscal year 1982 and eliminated in fiscal year 1983. House and Senate Appropriations Committees have shown some concern that in fiscal year 1982, funds should be targeted for specialties in short supply, disadvantaged students, and training in geriatrics and child psychiatry. Traditionally, support for clinical training has been centered in Congress; thus, much depends on the actions of Congress if we are to expect continued clinical training support (APA, 1981).

Continuing education gets only token funding. The high fees charged for such important educational programs are unrealistic when it comes to attracting ethnic minorities, other poorer paid professionals, and "other mental health workers" to the field. Mental health agencies themselves provide the support for many of the continuing education programs they conduct, but these costs are then passed on to those who pay for the services, which results in higher prices for mental health care. Serious questions must be raised about the use of funds intended for service delivery being used to pay for education. In recent years, there has been a strong trend to separate mental health training budgets from service budgets and to place training funds in the budgets of educational programs. However, reductions in training program budgets are forcing reexamination of this policy (President's Commission, 1978b).

The same task panel report summarizes how the problem of obtaining satisfactory data on the supply, education, and distribution of personnel has severely hampered national planning. The result is that we are placed in a situation of having to work with disjointed information from several sources–nonuniform, overlapping, and noncomplementary data–rather than in a coordinated system. For example, staffing data for health and mental health facilities come from the NIMH and from National Center for Health statistics, licensure data exist for only some professions, the American Medical Association monitors the data for the supply of medical doctors, and professional associations maintain a roster of their members and may conduct surveys of their activities, place of work, and salaries. Staffing data are weak on differentiating the various categories of paraprofessionals and cannot provide information on professionals in private practice or those employed in nontraditional mental health facilities. Licensure data provide little more than a head count and are incomplete for those professions such as psychology and social work where licensure is not universally mandatory for practice. Surveys by professional societies usually include only their own members. Data on geographic distribution are gross and insufficient for planning purposes, and little is known of the pattern of multiple employment that exists for many professionals. These data are needed for a rational assessment of mental health personnel needs and supply. It is believed that while states and localities can assist in the collection of these data, federal support and direction are essential for consistency and comprehensiveness, and as a vital part of national identification of needs and program planning. The NIMH should devote more attention and resources to the development of a data system and use it as an integral part of its policy making and program evaluation.

APHA'S ROLE

Let us now take a brief look at the APHA's role in assisting the manpower goals for mental health during the past 25 years. Prior to 1963, landmark year of President John F. Kennedy's strong support for community mental health and retardation services, the APHA endorsed the expansion of programs for training professional health personnel for service in mental retardation work, supported increased participation by public health agencies in mental health programs, urged the Public Health Service (PHS) to make training grants available to institutions for research workers in the field of mental health, and encouraged federal, state, and local governments to base and extend mental health and mental retardation care in general hospitals and health care facilities. During the next decade, the APHA strongly urged government to reduce the negative effects of practiced racism in the health and mental health fields by awarding increased training stipends to institutions of higher learning and professional schools that were producing greater percentages of Black health professionals, and to continue to do so until complete parity was achieved. Shortages in those of Spanish heritage were recognized when the APHA recommended and supported health legislation categorically oriented toward improving the skills and increasing the numbers of bilingual and bicultural ancillary health care workers. It is apparent that through its many resolutions, the APHA's role has been effective.

A review of manpower uses in mental health would not be complete without mention of some continuing, unresolved problems in mental health. It is remarkable that the statistics about mental health problems in the United States do not change significantly over time. For example, estimates are that mental disturbances afflict about 10 percent of the population, mental retardation 3.5 percent, alcoholism about 10 percent, and drug dependencies large proportions (the exact percentage is not usually reported). Just as remarkable is the fact that the mental health system manages to remain separated from the general health care system. Regier et al. (1978) have shown that the majority of mental patients rely heavily on the general medical sector for mental health care. The two systems are separated conceptually and physically; that is, the places for treatment of mental disorders are most often set apart physically from places offering care for physical ills. The mental health system as well remains separated from several other systems that are closely and equally concerned with mental health, such as the welfare system, the education system at all levels, the vocational system at almost all levels, and the judicial system. This isolation of mental health services from the other systems is deeply rooted and may reflect the historical fact that care of the mentally ill, unlike most other fields of personal health services, has been largely a public function in the United States. However, it does not require much research to discover that similar fragmentation, in the form of uncoordinated, categorical, and segmented programs, exists in the predominantly privately funded general health care system (see Coleman, Chapter 12, this volume).

It seems that public sponsorship of programs should produce the opposite of what has just been described. We would expect to see more coordination and integration, less duplication, fewer deficiencies in providing needed programs, and fewer piecemeal patchwork efforts, especially in view of decreasing funds and other sparse resources. Yet numerous overlapping and pyramidal agencies in complex bureaucratic structures at all levels of government—local, regional, state, and national—continue to exist. This problem remains one of the major puzzles in the provision of care delivery to the psychologically disordered in this nation (Roemer et al., 1975).

CONCLUSION

In sum, we still lack an effective comprehensive health care delivery system for all of humankind's ailments, physical and psychological, as well as treatment programs for every person, regardless of ability to pay. Meanwhile, we continue to have fragmented programs, and providers offer little in the way of responsibility or accountability. Discriminatory practices in service delivery are rampant, along with abject poverty and a demonstrated inability to cope with and tolerate new groups and problems that have emerged as a result of improved technology.

In recent decades, numerous ideas for bringing general health care to our nation's entire population have been proposed, and they in turn have raised two important questions, if only by their omission. First, the proposals generally have failed to provide sufficiently for prescription drugs, dental care for children, and outpatient psychiatric care. Second, while there have been improvements, racial discriminatory practices have long been major barriers to health and mental health care. Grave problems are still with us: job discrimination and poor schooling together limit employment opportunities; low income levels which, when combined with discriminatory practices, diminish the opportunity to attain good health and mental health education and care (Penn & Penn, 1976).

Since we know what the problems are, are well aware of this nation's responsibility to resolve them, perhaps our nation's main problem is the absence of a model, a model of a human community in which inequities in care delivery and in "caring" as it relates to personnel power cannot exist. What would this human community look like? How would it be defined? In describing this community, I will borrow from a definition by social psychologist Robert Dentler (1968). This community would be a nexus, or a point in a terrain where society, culture, and individuals meet, and where social interaction would be repeated frequently. It would provide an organization of social activities in ways that give individuals local access to all that is essential for day-to-day living, and where a person could find all or most of the economic, political, religious, and familial institutions around which people group to cooperate, to compete, or to engage in conflict. It would have a range of functions that has an equivalent in the range of social positions required of a modern community, and it would contain a population of each kind of person our society or culture knows for as long as the categories repeated themselves through the successive lives of the members of the community. For example, a grouping or ghetto of senior citizens, single parents, or Black people or Jewish people is by this definition not a community. This community may be larger than a city, a state, or neighborhood. We cannot stop the drawing of its boundaries until all of the foregoing requirements have been satisfied. This community includes all of us. It would provide for the needs and demands of every person, since this would be a necessary requirement for its survival. Finally, it would make every person responsible and accountable for the community's continued existence.

In her presidential message to the annual meeting of the APHA in 1980, Dr. June Jackson Christmas stated that "in order to have a whole body, we need both a head and a heart, and . . . if we are to have a whole society we need an agenda and a message." The community described herein, I believe, has the proper agenda and message: survival and caring. It would demand, as well as encourage, the various mental health and health disciplines and other agencies to communicate effectively and plan functionally as we strive to reach our society's and this human community's explicit goals.

The concerns addressed in this chapter were manpower and training—their development, distribution, and financial support—both of which are central to the establishment of a community that is survival-oriented and caring, which has both "a head and a heart . . . a message and an agenda." The degree to which the severe funding restrictions and cutbacks proposed by our current government administrators are achieved, will, to a similar extent, limit opportunities to improve on our society's goals of health and welfare for all of its citizens. Article I,

Section 8 of the U.S. Constitution wisely states that "the Congress shall have the power to . . . provide for the common defense and general welfare," thus including public health as well as psychological well-being. Since that time, other governmental officials have seen fit to speak to the issue of promoting mental health. Some selected statements follow:

> It seems that there is nothing new today except the remarkability that old problems continue to exist today, and that approaches to resolution may be more complex than today's human kind can fathom.
>
> –Unknown, early 1900s

> Disease is largely a removable evil. It continues to afflict humanity, not only because of incomplete knowledge of its causes and lack of adequate individual and public hygiene, but also because it is extensively fostered by harsh economic and industrial conditions and by wretched housing in congested communities. These conditions and consequently the diseases which spring from them can be removed by better social organization. No duty of society, acting through its governmental agencies, is paramount to this obligation to attack the removable causes of disease. The duty of leading this attack and bringing home to public opinion the fact that the community can buy its own health protection is laid upon all health officers, organizations and individuals interested in public health movements. For the provision of more and better facilities for the protection of the public health must come in the last analysis through the education of public opinion so that the community shall vividly realize both its needs and its powers.
>
> –Hermann M. Biggs
Monthly Bulletin
New York City Health
Department
October 1911

> The United States has the economic resources, the organizing ability and the technical experience to solve our unnecessary health care problems, that is, the tremendous amounts of preventable physical pain and mental anguish, needless deaths, economic inefficiency, and social waste.
>
> –Ray L. Wilburn
Secretary of the Interior, 1932

cancerous racial discrimination inflicts immeasurable human and social costs on a large number of U.S. citizens. . . . Discrimination in education, training, employment, and union membership impedes development of human resources, reduces efficiency and slows the economy while simultaneously altering inequitably the distribution of the fruits of economic progress.

—A. Celebrezzi
DHEW Secretary, 1963

It is important that we, today, take on whatever the responsibilities are for continuing our efforts to provide for our mental health now and in the future. In our role as mental health professionals, we must make the most of every opportunity that places and maintains the survival of humankind among our nation's highest priorities.

References

APA Report. *Status report on the federal budget as it affects psychology, and social and behavioral research, training and services.* Washington, DC: Author, December, 1981.

BASS, R. D. *CMHC staffing: Who minds the store.* DHEW Publication No. 78-686. Washington, DC: Government Printing Office, 1978.

DENTLER, R. A. *American community problems.* New York: McGraw-Hill, 1968.

HAUSMAN, K. *Psychiatric News,* September 1980.

Joint Commission on Mental Illness and Health. *Action for mental health.* New York: Basic Books, 1961.

National Institute for Mental Health. *Staffing patterns in mental health facilities.* Publication No. 5034. Washington, DC: Government Printing Office, 1970.

PENN, N. E., & PENN, B. P. The role of the federal government in promoting general welfare. In E. J. Lieberman (Ed.), *Mental health: The public health challenge.* Washington, DC: APHA, 1976.

The President's Commission on Mental Health. *Report to the President, Vol. I: New directions for personnel.* Washington, DC: Government Printing Office, 1978. (a)

The President's Commission on Mental Health. *Report to the President, Vol. II: Task panel report on mental health personnel.* Washington, DC: Government Printing Office, 1978. (b)

REGIER, D. A., GOLDBERG, I. G., & TAUBE, C. A. The de facto in the U.S. mental health service system: A public health perspective. *Archives of General Psychiatry,* 1978, *35,* 685-693.

ROEMER, R., KRAMER, C., & FRINK, J. *Planning urban health services.* New York: Springer, 1975.

ROSENSTEIN, M., & TAUBE, C. *Staffing of mental health facilities, United States, 1976.* NIMH Publication No. 78-522. Washington, DC: Government Printing Office, 1978.

TAUBE, C. *Staffing of mental health facilities, United States, 1972.* NIMH Publication No. 74-28. Washington, DC: Government Printing Office, 1974.

TAUBE, C. *Staffing of mental health facilities, United States, 1974.* NIMH Publication No. 76-308. Washington, DC: Government Printing Office, 1976.

Chapter 8

CHANGING PRACTICES IN PERSONNEL PREPARATION AND USE

DWIGHT W. RIEMAN

In her remarkable book, *I'm Dancing As Fast As I can,* Barbara Gordon (1979) vividly describes her experience with the "mental health establishment." During several years she managed to survive encounters with 20 therapists, two mental hospitals, countless medications, and staggering bills. She was diagnosed: schizophrenic, manic depressive, cyclothymic, borderline psychotic, agitated depressive, hysterical, and just plain neurotic. These, she says, were just "a few of the labels this broad brush of scientific endeavor pasted on me. I have been over medicated, over analyzed and under analyzed. I have been given suicidal advice. But somehow along the way, I have met a few wise and tender people. Too few."

Gordon describes psychiatry as a "fragile science." Although her criticism is mostly about psychiatry in the private sector, she also indicts much of the mental health system, private and public. Her book has important implications–past and current–for mental health programming, training, and use of personnel.

I might add that in addition to mental health, some of the "hard sciences" may also be "fragile." I refer to applications (or misapplications) of physics, chemistry, and biology in relation to energy development, nuclear power management, waste disposal, and patenting of living organisms, to name a few. This note of pessimism does not, by and large, characterize what I will say about progress and changing practices during the past 25 years. There have been many outstanding developments, but also many problems in the use and training of mental health personnel.

PROGRESS–DEFINED

Progress considerations as discussed here relate primarily to quality of services and education efforts, and only in a lesser way to increases in volume. Did the effort improve services to individuals, families, and communities? Did it turn out better prepared practitioners? Was interagency and interdisciplinary activity improved? Was there a loop of feedback (practice-education-practice? Did we look at the results of our personnel and training efforts and make necessary corrections? How well did we build and share knowledge? Did we contribute (or should we) to "quality of life" in the community, nation, and world? The recent Love Canal exposures sharpen the importance of this question. Love Canal brought not only profound physical problems and suffering to many people but also significant increases in marital problems, family problems, suicides, and depressions (National Broadcasting Corporation, 1980).

PROGRESS–PERSONNEL

Volume

The supply of professionals in mental health and related settings during the past quarter-century has more than tripled. From 1955 to 1978, the number of psychiatrists increased from 10,600 to 28,000; psychologists from 13,500 to 47,000; social workers (NASW members) from 20,000 to 76,000. Psychiatric nurse figures for 1955 are not available, but their numbers in 1976 were 48,000 (Vischi et al., 1980; President's Commission, 1978).

Data on psychiatrists through 1960 include APA membership plus filled psychiatric residencies; thereafter, data also include nonmembers of the APA who report a psychiatric specialization to the American Medical Association. Data on psychologists include membership in the APA. Approximately 30 percent of all psychologists are in clinical or counseling and guidance psychology. Many others are in mental health-related areas. Of all social workers, 20-25 percent are estimated to be in psychiatric or mental health areas.

The completeness and reliability of data on personnel leave much to be desired. Here are some examples from social work, as reported by Loavenbruck (1979):

> In doing social work manpower research, analysis and projections, one is concerned primarily with supply and demand indicators. To date, our data on supply of social work manpower is limited, fragmented, uneven, based on many questionable guessed estimates. No one federal agency or national organization collects comprehensive data on the social work manpower pool. There are numerous fields in which social workers are employed which tend to serve as a barrier to comprehensive data collection. Different federal agencies have very different reasons for collecting (or not collecting) data on social work manpower in these many fields. There are many different levels (professional and pre-professional) of social workers, which further confounds the data collection picture. There are also many different and often conflicting operational definitions of social workers, some professionally inspired, some of a quasi legal nature, and still others reflecting common public usage, e.g., social worker vs. social services worker vs. welfare worker. Our professional association collects data only on its membership and that represents, at best, a slice of the total picture. Not since 1960 has any national data been collected on the educational levels of social service workers: e.g., in 1960 about 2/3 of the workers had no graduate study while about 17% had an MSW or equivalent and a like proportion had some graduate work. We know from council statistics that the number of MSW's has exploded through the 60's and 70's.

Dollars for mental health services have also increased markedly: "In the late 1950's the direct cost of mental illness was estimated to be $1.7 billion a year. By 1976, the direct costs of providing mental health services was about $17 billion, approximately 12% of all health costs. Over 50% of these expenditures were for services provided in nursing homes and also public mental hospitals" (President's Commission, 1978).

Broadened Use of Paraprofessional, Nonprofessional, and Indigenous Workers

There was an explosion in the numbers and use of these personnel during the 25-year period from 1955 to 1978. This is a clear indicator of progress, not only because it extended the labor pool but also because each of these groups made unique and distinct contributions to services. I have had occasion to work with many of them in a training capacity, and I have also had opportunity to observe their work in many settings. One of these was in a demonstration project of social services for residents of public housing in rural areas. Indigenous workers and paraprofessionals were used extensively and successfully in this project (University of Missouri, 1979a).

No known data about paraprofessionals are available for 1955, but 1977-78 figures indicate that there were at least 150,000 in mental health, alcohol, and drug abuse programs. Of these, about 145,000 (FTE) were patient care staff in mental health facilities. Fully 90 percent were employed in inpatient settings (Vischi et al., 1980).

In all, 30,000 paraprofessionals were trained in over 500 programs in both two- and four-year college sequences. Graduates increased from 4,000 in 1970 to 10,000 in 1977, with a projection of 12,500 in 1980 (President's Commission, 1978).

Paraprofessionals perform many useful tasks in a variety of settings as psychiatric aides and technicians in intake, outreach, after care, and more recently in community care programs for the chronically mentally disabled.

The nonprofessional may be an extension of the professional—an aide who can reduce the burden on the professional worker. Reif and Riessman (1965) refer to them as the "ubiquitous" nonprofessionals who are often recruited from the ranks of those with the same social background, attitudes, values, and so forth as the professional (housewives, college students, and so on). Sometimes the role as aide to the professional eclipses their value as aide to the client.

The indigenous nonprofessional, in contrast, is from the "neighborhood," often poor, a member of a minority group, and with a common background, language, ethnic origin, and style with clients from the same neighborhood or community. He or she not only complements the professional by taking over lesser tasks but can also fulfill new ones. Sometimes, however, with poor supervision and inadequate training, the indigenous worker becomes "contaminated" with what is perceived to be the agency's point of view regarding the poor or low-income client; for example, being thought of as "lazy" or "not wanting to help themselves" (Reiff & Riessman, 1965).

Even though indigenous and other nonprofessionals are no panacea, they have highly important contributions to make—if the tasks are carefully selected, if the workers are carefully screened before their employment (attitudes, values, capacity to develop, and so forth), and if there is time and motivation for careful orientation, inservice training, and supervision.

Allied Mental Health Professionals

Another example of enlarging the personnel pool during the period was the addition of a wide range of other professionals who now make up about 12 percent (FTE) of patient care staff. These include pastoral counselors, counseling and guidance personnel, occupational therapists, vocational counselors, special education teachers, recreation therapists, marriage counselors, and art therapists. For example, there are over 1200 registered music therapists (President's Commission, 1978).

The Davenports (1979) describe important recent additions of allied personnel, including students and graduates in "people-oriented" disciplines assigned to work in energy-impacted communities (boom towns): personnel from anthropology, recreation, adult education, law, and communications.

Extended Discovery and Application of Board Member Talents

With the organization of almost 700 community mental health centers since 1963, a large number of board members have also emerged. Although the volume of members is not known, it does represent many thousands of talented people. The use of board members varies widely, and the potential for their contribution is still far from realized. But the past 15 years have seen encouraging expansion in creative use of board members, going far beyond assignments in traditional, often menial kinds of tasks, to responsible participation with staff in the design, operation, and evaluation of community mental health programs.

Increased Flexibility in Role and Function—Professional and Organizational

A healthy, although stressful and by no means completed development, has been in role flexibility among professionals and organizations. Sacred and traditional turfs have been successfully challenged. Boundaries for service vary by discipline, and opportunities for special use of individual talents were expanded greatly.

Some will recall a number of years ago the endless discussions of disciplinary uniqueness. There is now, fortunately, less preoccupation with "what is our unique contribution?" and more attention to what is the individual, family, or community need, and who is best able and available to meet it? There has been positive competition between disciplines, centers, hospitals, and community agencies. There has also been destructive competition resulting in poor services and often denial of service choices to individuals.

Drug selections and supervision remain the responsibility of the physician. The rest of us have been spared that burden. It has become in many instances an "albatross." Too often, drugs are easy and mechanical substitutes for human care, with resulting addiction and nonrecovery.

One example of increased flexibility in personnel use is the change in administration of mental health services. Ten years ago, most centers and hospitals were administered by psychiatrists. Since then, other disciplines have increasingly assumed this responsibility. In 1971 psychiatrists administered 55 percent of federally funded community mental health centers. In 1976, this figure dropped to 30 percent. Psychologist administrators increased from 16 percent in 1971 to 21 percent in 1976. In 1971 social work represented 17 percent of administrators. In 1976 they administered 31 percent of the centers.

"Other" disciplines comprised 5 percent of center administrators in 1971. This grew to 15 percent in 1976 (NIMH, 1978).

There has been a disturbing decline in the number of staff psychiatrists and trainees in mental health centers. Although changes in administration from predominance by psychiatrists is, to me, an encouraging development, the loss of staff psychiatrists and trainees is a serious problem.

A related problem is the relatively small number of psychiatrists specializing in child psychiatry—only about 2,800, when 11,000 are needed. Each year, 200 complete training. For the other end of the age spectrum, there are only a handful of psychiatrists who specialize in problems of the aged, yet by the year 2000 approximately 25 percent of the population will be over 65 (President's Commission, 1978).

Dr. Henry Foley, administrator of the Health Resources Administration, has stated that "medical students are discouraged from going into psychiatry because other areas of practice are more lucrative." One solution he suggests is that medical schools train more physicians in psychiatric diagnostic skills and "not turn them into psychiatrists as we did 20 years ago through NIMH special project grants" (ADAMHA News, 1980a).

Whether you agree with this suggestion or not, the loss of psychiatrists from mental health settings and the failure to attract young psychiatrists in significant numbers are very serious problems. Obviously, we need to know much more about the reasons for the loss before anything very productive can be done.

Increased Effectiveness and Utilization of Person Power Through Consultation

There has been encouraging growth in consultation knowledge and skills development, numbers of mental health personnel involved in consultation activities, and in training efforts to improve this important pursuit. In 1955 one could count the number of references on one hand. Today there are hundreds, and the problem becomes one of selecting the most appropriate and useful ones. Two very important contributions to annotation and cataloging are: (1) "Consultation in Mental Health and

Related Fields: A Reference Guide" (Mannino, 1969) and (2) "The Practice of Mental Health Consultation" (Mannino, et al., 1975).

The monograph, "Consultation in Social Work Practice," is, among some others, a classic reference for all disciplines. Why it was allowed to go out of print so quickly is a mystery. Perhaps it was ahead of its time in 1963 when consultation was just beginning to catch on (Rapoport, 1963). The insistence on consultation and educational activities, within the range of necessary services to qualify for federal funding, is one kind of federal "encroachment" that has been very positive.

The task of promoting and protecting the mental and physical health of the population requires imaginative variation and enlargement of present methods. Even though important gains have been made during this past quarter-century, the struggle must continue with decisions about accomplishing the most with the fewest people and the least effort.

We must be concerned not only with those who are sick, but also with keeping healthy people well. It seems safe to assume that in the next decade there will not be enough mental health specialists to help even all of the sick people, not to mention those troubled with simpler, "garden variety" kinds of problems.

Looking at only one very vulnerable population, for example, it is modestly estimated that there are at least 500,000 cases of child abuse and neglect per year. Somewhere between 2,000 and 5,000 children are killed by their parents each year. In 1975, 655,000 children under age 18 were admitted to an organized mental health facility, and yet this represents only 1 percent of all children in the United States and only a small percentage of those requiring mental health intervention (ADAMHA News, 1980b).

A further argument for extending consultation and education activities is that even if there were more specialists, many nonspecialized personnel are in more natural and strategic positions—often during times of crisis—to help those with whom they are in frequent contact. With traditional diagnostic and treatment approaches, we but dent the total problem. Mental health professions need allies to carry out large-scale preventive, education, and treatment activities. Consultation and education can help to develop and extend the skills of our allies (Rieman, 1967).

The influence of opinion leaders on the patterns and funding of human services, including mental health, is well established, but consultation and training efforts aimed at the enlightment of such leaders have received relatively little attention.

Unfortunately, even though the importance of consultation, in relation to extending services to troubled people through use of helping allies, has been reasonably well accepted, it still represents a very small percentage of total mental health center activity. Worse yet, with the budget crunch and an emphasis on more and easier reimbursable services, consultation and educational activities are on the decline nationally. This is a particularly acute problem with community mental health center "graduates." These are the 50 percent of the 668 centers no longer receiving basic NIMH staffing and operations grant support.

This "abandoned" graduate group needs funding for services to high-risk population groups and for nonreimbursable services, such as consultation and education, prevention, and evaluation. "Loss of federal funding has meant a shift toward the medical model, direct clinical and in-patient services, a subversion of center ideology, and pressures to limit services and to engage in other 'survival' behaviors" (ADAMHA News, 1980c).

Increasing Personnel Effectiveness Through Coordination and Collaboration of Mental Health and Related Disciplines and Services

The task through the years (and still a chronic problem) is not only one of recruiting additional personnel, nor of adding more and different kinds of services, but that of making the most efficient use of *existing* person power and services through effective coordination and collaborative patterns of work between mental health and care-giving staffs. For the purposes of this chapter, a working definition of coordination/collaboration is: (1) the working together of mental health and community care-giving agencies and staff in the provision of services to the mentally ill and their families, and (2) the design, administration, and revision of mental health and community care-giving programs in such ways as to promote and encourage active intra- and interagency coordination/collaboration.

Coordination and collaboration, often loosely used terms, have in common the concept of rationally planned and executed services. The two terms and processes are related but different. Coordination is particularly applicable to interagency planning and administration of services to a segment of the population, whereas collaboration is more attuned to interagency delivery of services to an individual or family. Coordination may be considered as a mutually agreed upon service pattern and content by a group of agencies, with a division of labor in the provision of services to designated population groups.

In collaborative service delivery, it may be assumed that coordination at interagency administrative levels already exists or is in process. It may also be assumed in the collaborative process that there is acceptance by all parties of a common diagnostic treatment plan, with a division of labor and accompanying agreement on priorities and goals for service to a given individual or family.

On the other hand, coordination may not be a preexisting condition, and one or a series of collaborative experiences and exercises may be necessary to develop coordination at program planning and administrative levels. Or, coordination at planning and administrative levels may be the preexisting condition that leads to effective interagency collaboration.

Since any absolute distinction between the two processes and precise and separate definitions of both are difficult and somewhat personal, the two are used together (and somewhat interchangeably) in the following look at interagency and interdisciplinary efforts.

Although some progress has been made in these efforts, it has not been steady. Indeed, we may now be in a period of regression or deterioration in coordination/collaborative efforts. Considerations in behalf of patient rights and confidentiality, though very important, have resulted all too often (for "survival" purposes) in little or no exchange of information within and between agencies. Actually, when the need is presented properly, most patients will encourage such exchange. "Helping with the hurt" is more important to them than "Who knows about my problem?"

The mentally ill and their families are frequently known to a variety of community services. Unfortunately, many times each service operates independently or without knowledge of another's operations. The patient, client, or student may be understood only as the probationer, the welfare recipient, the school failure, the religiously mixed up person, the psychiatrically disturbed, or the person with a physical health problem. They or their family may be all of these, and as many agencies or services may be working on certain aspects of the total problem according to their own unique function, without a unitary view of the person or of effective approaches in serving him or her as an individual within a family and a community. The various services may, in fact, be working in direct contradiction or opposition to what others are attempting. The individual or family problem may also be one of such enormity, or the particular agency services may be so restricted in function, that other problems or individuals within the family unit may be overlooked, with consequent failure to provide early, preventive services.

When an individual or a family is served by mental health and community care-giving staff, and possibly by one or more private practitioners, it would be well to look at the overall problem and ask of each agency, staff worker, and practitioner: "Who does what, why, and when?" "Is a coordinator or 'captain' of the helping team needed?"

Additional coordination/collaboration concerns include:

(1) Extent of awareness on the part of care-giving personnel when mental illness is developing in a family they are serving. If awareness is present, how freely and effectively do they call on mental health professionals for direct services and/or consultation?

(2) Sensitivity and methods of care-giving personnel regarding their attempts to help a family when a developing mental illness is recognized. What, if any, help do they seek from mental professionals: direct services to the patient and family, consultation, methods of coordination/collaboration?

The following are offered as examples of problems in coordination/collaboration. First, for mental health professionals:

(1) Will the mental health professional accept in a practical operative

way the concept of the "extended team" in services to patients and families?

(2) Does the MH professional regard collaborative/coordinative process as worthwhile? ("Are the other team participants really any good and/or will their active involvement in planning and implementation of services really be of any value?")
(3) Will the professional accept a care-giver with less training or specialization in a field other than mental health as a peer in the coordinating/collaborative team?
(4) Will the professional take the time and make the effort to involve "collaborators" or simply resort to an independent plan of action that represents only mental health staff/facility?
(5) Will one discipline (within the mental health facility) accept representatives from other disciplines as peers in the design and implementation of service plans?

About related agency personnel and care-givers, the following questions are raised:

(1) Are they intimidated by those with more extensive training or by representatives of mental health professionals whom they may regard as "head shrinkers"?
(2) Will they wonder (with resulting inhibitions), "Are they going to read my mind?"
(3) Will they feel inadequate and not offer suggestions or ideas, thinking that they may be criticized for them?
(4) Are they already so overburdened with work demands that attempts to work in collaborative ways with mental health staff may be regarded as an impossible burden?
(5) Can they accept the idea that quite often an expenditure of time in behalf of a patient or family may result ultimately in a saving of time, or at least in better return in terms of service results?
(6) Will the care-giver be so unsure or uncertain because of feelings of inadequacy that he or she would rather accept a "plan" presented by the mental health "expert" as "superior" to one in whose design he or she may play a part?

For both mental health professionals and community care-giving personnel, the following questions and concerns are presented:

(1) Can they effectively define their individual and group goals in work with patients and families?

(2) Can they accept the need to make interagency and intra- and interprofessional coordination a dynamic effort?
(3) Can both mental health and community care-giving personnel view family and individual needs on a long-term basis?
(4) Can they understand and accept the need to know one another as people to work together effectively?

Following many years of struggles with coordination/collaboration problems in varied service, planning, consultation, and educational efforts, I would offer the following as some very elementary and basic requirements for effective intra- and interagency coordination and collaboration:

(1) Acceptance at all staff levels of the importance of coordination and collaboration in service delivery, program planning, and administration of services;
(2) clearly defined service functions and responsibilities (and understanding of these) within service units/agencies;
(3) effective mutual understanding and agency intercommunication regarding the nature and scope of services and responsibilities; and
(4) opportunities for staff within service units and among agencies to get to know one another as people (not just names, addresses, or phone numbers), and to reconcile feelings and attitudes that may interfere with communication and functioning.

New Demands, Stresses, and Opportunities for Mental Health Personnel

Disasters–Natural and Man-Made. Examples are threats to mental health from storms, floods, tornadoes, and the recent Mt. St. Helens eruptions. Love Canal and Three-Mile Island had devastating effects. Mass fear still exists. Hundreds left the areas. The total impact, as well as what mental health services were provided, and their effects, await further study.

Chemical spills from derailed railroad cars last year in Sturgeon, Missouri, had serious effects on the mental and physical health of many, particularly the elderly and other poor persons living near the tracks. This experience also awaits further investigation of how mental health persons might help alleviate suffering.

The recent riots in Miami point up the importance of involving knowledgeable mental health personnel in prevention and control activities.

Still other examples of man-made "disasters" of almost epidemic proportions are abused children and adults, including rape victims.

Boom Towns. In their new book on the subject, the Davenports (1980) describe a stressful fact of life for many people, especially those residing in the energy-rich American West. They underline the unhappy fact that "our ability to extract and process mineral riches is not matched by our ability to deal with the social consequences and human costs of rapid growth and development."

In the same book, Weisz cites Gillette, Wyoming, and its 1974-78 boom, marked by a 101 percent increase in admissions to the local mental health center and a 601 percent increase in admissions to the state hospital, while during the same period the county population increased 62 percent (Davenport & Davenport, 1980: 1).

Fortunately, some foresighted professors from the University of Wyoming, with the help of a social work education grant from the National Institute of Mental Health, were able to intervene with "boom town" problems through the Wyoming Human Services Project. They developed innovative training procedures for social work and related students in human services to prepare them for both planning and direct services in energy-impacted communities. The training and educational efforts also resulted in the production of a reservoir of personnel to provide ongoing services to communities beyond the student field training experiences.

These efforts are exemplary and represent legitimate "quality of life" concerns for mental health personnel. The projects, books, and other writings about it are significant contributions to knowledge-building in the pioneering areas of stress prevention and control.

MBO, GOSS, Cost Effectiveness, and Other "Fads." Mental health and other human services personnel have experienced a plethora of procedures to improve program and worker effectiveness. Management by Objective, Goal-Oriented Social Services, and now cost effectiveness are illustrative of a few of these. Programs are sometimes shaped by their excellence in financial planning, with disproportionate attention to needs for services to people. There have been recent attempts to apply profit-oriented business techniques to community mental health centers, some of which are inappropriate for human service endeavors. Examples are given in a timely paper presented by Lebedun and Samuels at the annual meeting of the National Council of Community Mental Health Centers, 1980.

The authors describe information systems to monitor staff activity and establish precise unit cost data with the goal of raising productivity levels. Such procedures are similar to industrial management techniques aimed at increased productivity per unit cost and the demonstrated relationship has not been documented in the delivery of human services. Although the monitoring process may improve apparent productivity, the increases may come at some cost, such as redirection of effort away from work responsibilities that may be more difficult to measure, e.g., quality, investment in activities that have longer-run payoffs, and improved cooperation with fellow employees.

Lebedun and Samuels (1980) state that community mental health is considered most productive when it reduces demand and consumption of services, as is true with welfare agencies and police and fire departments, all of which have as a goal the reduction of social disorder. Reducing the demand for services is dissimilar to the functioning of private business, whose success and revenue are measured by increased demands for products/services. "How many businesses invest large amounts of effort and financial resources showing people how to avoid the need for their product?" The authors rightly question "the unqualified application of private, productivity-oriented business approaches to a public human service endeavor."

Services to Minorities. There was considerable effort, but with questionable results, to improve services during the past decade for racial groups, the elderly, children, and the poor. In addition to further innovations for improved services to these groups, attention needs to be given to services for two new groups in our midst: Southeast Asians and Cubans. These groups not only offer new service challenges but also the opportunity for contributions from mental health personnel in community organization and advocacy activities.

Community Care for the Chronically Mentally Ill. The chronically mentally disabled, a long-neglected population in hospital back wards during earlier years, have been rediscovered as a very neglected population on the back streets of our cities.

There was a dramatic reduction of hospital populations from more than 500,000 in the mid-1950s to recent figures of under 200,000. Although this was a very significant development, one of the all-too-frequent consequences was inferior care or no care at all for many in the community.

The task panel on deinstitutionalization of the President's Commission on Mental Health gave high priority to the development of community support services and housing for this neglected minority. The urgency, scope, and timeliness of the panel's recommendations are highlighted in the following excerpts from their report:

> The chronically mentally disabled are severely and persistently ill. These are the people who are, have been or might have been in earlier times, residents of large mental institutions. They constitute that subgroup of the mentally ill for whom societal rejection has been, and is, most acute.
>
> The chronically mentally disabled are a minority within minorities. They are the most stigmatized of the mentally ill. They are politically and economically powerless and rarely speak for themselves. Their stigma is multiplied, since disproportionate numbers among them are people who are also elderly, poor, or members of racial or ethnic minority groups. They are the totally disenfranchised among us.
>
> Deinstitutionalization, ostensibly intended to assist the chronically mentally disabled by taking or keeping them out of large, understaffed, public mental hospitals and permitting them to be cared for in the community has fallen short of its goal. Unfortunately, deinstitutionalization has too often occurred without adequate planning.
>
> Stigma does not stop when they leave the hospital; it follows them wherever they go. The community rejection that may have contributed to their hospitalization is only increased when these patients are returned to the community without the supportive services they so desperately need [President's Commission, 1978].

Although certainly not a new minority, the rediscovery of this population does present new challenges and opportunities for mental health personnel. Mental health professionals are not readily available, however, to serve them, and in many instances paraprofessionals and indigenous workers can provide very appropriate and needed services if adequate supervision, orientation, and training are available from professionals.

Traditional clinical approaches are often inappropriate and sometimes even destructive for many of the chronically disabled. What is needed are highly individualized living and service arrangements that are the least restrictive, most humane, relevant, and varied according to the diverse and complex needs of this special clientele.

Although community mental health centers are required by the 1975 amendments to provide services for this population, there seems to be little evidence that such services are being offered in any significant volume. Centers, working cooperatively with other organizations, public and private, can offer much through diagnostic and emergency services, consultation and training for paraprofessionals, and in back-up support to many groups serving the mentally disabled.

Self-Help Groups—Friends or Foes

The development of such groups has been conspicuous since World War II, with a great period of expansion during the 1960s. New groups emerge as people continue to need, give, and seek help from others. The following typology of groups from Katz and Bender (1976: 9) is offered in highly abbreviated form:

(1) self-fulfillment or personal growth–example, Recovery Incorporated;
(2) social advocacy–example, welfare rights organizations;
(3) alternative patterns for living–examples, Gay Liberation, communes;
(4) "rock bottom"–example, Synanon;
(5) "mixed"–having characteristics of two or more of the above.

Katz (1977: 1257-1260) writes that after some 20 years of neglect, social practitioners are now beginning to take self-help groups seriously, with the realization that they will endure and that they have many useful aspects. He cautions, however, that their widespread emergence poses both opportunities and dangers for the professional community. One danger is seeing them as all the same or as a panacea for professional failures. Another is to give them powers they do not possess. He suggests that perhaps the greatest danger is "that of co-optation of the groups by professionals, which would defeat the groups' purposes and destroy their distinctive character."

Tensions do exist between mental health professionals and self-help groups. Serious study is needed as to why these tensions exist and how to make them creative rather than destructive.

Personnel Abuse—Burnout

Burnout occurs with alarming frequency at all professional levels. The literature is flooded with definitions, sources of the problem, and "solutions." Numbers of burnout workshops have ballooned.

Burnout is not a new phenomenon, and certainly not one unique to mental health. What is new and healthy is the increased recognition that the problem does exist in serious proportions, and that it can happen to any and all of us. It is no longer a mark of disgrace or weakness when burnout occurs.

We are, however, coming to recognize all too slowly the importance of investing money, time, and talent, both on and off the job, to try to prevent or alleviate the problem. It is highly complex, whether self-imposed, administratively imposed, systems-imposed, or the result of a combination of these and other factors. Burnout is obviously a very individual problem. What may be stressful for some in the workplace may be stimulating and creative for others.

There are few good "package" solutions to burnout. To be helpful, workshops must offer strongly individualized approaches through which persons and organizations may find solutions consistent with the uniqueness of circumstances, personal and organizational, both during and following the workshop. We need to carefully analyze the after-effects of workshop experiences.

I will not add to the mounting literature on burnout. However, from a recent retreat for staff of a mental health center, I will share some simple, human thoughts and suggestions. Burnout was an important topic.

I served as consultant on retreat design and also as "facilitator" during the one-day session. It was attended by almost three-fourths of the total staff at all levels. Administration participated actively in the design and as participants.

From summary remarks at the close of the retreat come these quotes on burnout:

- Set up a system whereby we as staff members can set up appointments with *other staff* of our choice for counseling when *we* need to talk to somebody. Limits perhaps, but maybe two hours of staff counseling a month.
- Unstructured staff time when we can just get together and sit and talk and get to know one another.
- We need positive strokes from ourselves and from administration. Somebody does a good job and we need to say: "Hey, you did a good job." But if we don't *know* what they're doing, we can't tell them that.
- Seems like we're all the targets–all the fingers are pointing inside. We need to point some fingers *outside.*
- *Distance*–we're all in the same office, or in the same building or around the block from each other, but we're thousands of miles apart.
- Contagious hilarity!
- Screwing off–we know that is good sometimes, but we need to know that others know it and even support it!
- We need a *sense of history* about our work and about this place.
- Who *is* my supervisor?
- I don't really know *what* my job is.
- I wish people would say "*hello*" to me, and not just talk to me when they want something from me. Please say "hello" to me.
- I make suggestions, and I ask questions. I get no response. Nothing happens. I don't get any recognition.
- There is more and more emphasis on *production* when I am already overworked. They don't listen to my data. I tell them how much I am doing, but they don't hear it, and they say work more.
- There seem to be rewards only for *paying* things. Money.
- Paper work has become more important than people work.

PROGRESS–TRAINING: BASIC PROFESSIONAL

Volume

The training budget of the NIMH in 1955 was $4.8 million. In 1960, it was $24.8 million. It reached a high of $120 million in 1969. Major emphasis was on basic education for the mental health professions.

In 1972, 44 percent of psychiatric residents, 28 percent of graduate clinical psychology students, 38 percent of master's-level psychiatric social work, students, and 90 percent of master's degree candidates in psychiatric nursing were receiving NIMH stipends. Since 1972, however, NIMH appropriations for training have become progressively lower, the number of stipends has been reduced, particularly in psychiatry, and faculty support for other professional departments has been drastically reduced (President's Commission, 1978).

A President's Commission Task Force has pointed out that decreasing federal support will result, among other things, in fewer numbers of poor and minority students "and graduate and professional schools may become the preserve of the upper middle classes, oriented toward private practice" (President's Commission, 1978).

Degrees awarded increased during the period 1960-76 for psychology (Ph.D.) from 773 to 2878; for social work (master's) from 2078 to 9080; for psychiatric nursing (master's) from 193 to 551 (1975); and for psychiatry (residents) from 3400 to 4864 (President's Commission, 1978).

Content—New Areas

There was marked expansion since 1955 in the array of new (or enriched) content areas, both in basic and continuing education. The following are examples: Crisis Intervention, Rural Mental Health, Consultation, Outreach, Work with Groups, Leadership, Childhood Development, Women, Minorities, Work with the Elderly, Behavioral Psychology, Holistic Approaches, Citizen Involvement, and Systems.

Interdisciplinary Efforts and Offerings

There has been some increase in the volume of graduate courses offered on a multidiscipline basis. However, improvement is needed both in the quality and number of such offerings. It is wasteful to duplicate courses when actual differences in content are slight. Some courses offered exclusively to a single discipline can, with some modification, be addressed to all the mental health professions, for example, "Community

Mental Health." The quality of such offerings is also enriched with an interdisciplinary student mix.

Adoption and Refinement of Generalist Approaches

One important development in social work education and practice is the expanded use of the generalist model. This emphasizes the problem to be solved rather than adherence to a given method (Rubin, 1979: 30).

At the University of Missouri School of Social Work, a generalist is defined as one who identifies and assesses social phenomena in their various systemic ramifications and, based on that assessment, differentially intervenes wherever it is efficient and effective to do so to produce legitimate social change. The uniquely different aspect of generalist practice is that it does not predetermine the scope nor focus on a problematic situation based on worker specialty. Potential interventions depend on resources which the worker has or can obtain (University of Missouri, 1978: 2-3).

Some Troubling Issues in Mental Health Education

Very compelling among these is the need for more and better "loops of feedback" about the results of education. Simply "linear" training of more and more persons is not enough. We need more knowledge of what they do and whether we have adequately prepared them for varied tasks in the field.

A related issue is the persistent gap between professional schools and practice agencies. Extended dialogues and cooperative research on mutual concerns are much needed.

There are continuing pressures to make professional schools into "technical schools," or in-service training units of mental health agencies. Schools must be responsive to service demands, yet they must maintain "purity" about their knowledge-building and knowledge-advancement missions. Otherwise, there is real danger of helping to perpetuate what may be bad practice systems by training people to maintain the status quo or do merely "patch up" work. Education should produce change, both individual and organizational–change, of course, for the better, if we know what that is.

With the current budget crunch at all levels, the loss of student training sites is already a harsh reality. One example described in a recent issue of the *NASW News* is the June 1980 demise of the outstanding social work program at Mt. Zion Hospital in San Francisco after "more than 30 years of training some of this country's best social workers." This was due to severe budget cuts because of the loss of federal, state, and local funds, exacerbated by the high rate of inflation and the reorientation of hospital priorities and commitments. NIMH training funds all but dried up, and Proposition 13 left its impact, with ceilings in Medi-Cal and cuts in Short-Doyle funding.

Hospitals in such crises lean toward rendering those services for which they can be assured reimbursement. Services to the poor are cut with a concomitant decrease in the number of social work jobs. "Ancillary" services are the least reimbursable and therefore the most dispensable.

This sad development poses a real threat to interdisciplinary gains made in service delivery and education. It further dramatizes the need for continued dialogue, cooperation, and mutual planning between service providers and educators.

Other pressing needs in education include: how to "glamorize" training for work with the chronically mentally ill, and increased attention to other disabled groups which are underserved, for example, the deaf, for whom almost no mental health services exist.

PROGRESS—CONTINUING EDUCATION

Definition

Viewed in its broadest terms, an "umbrella"-type definition of continuing education would be those offerings beyond the graduate degree, including staff development, in-service training, and adult education of many kinds. This definition includes all education endeavors beyond those usually considered appropriate for entrance into a mental health profession or occupation.

To look more precisely at different kinds of continuing education within the broad category, we might say that *in-service training* is agency-based: staff are the principal targets, and primary focus is on the rudiments of their present jobs.

Although staff do learn new skills in in-service training, transferability of skills and knowledge is limited, as is advancement of the profession.

Staff development has many similarities to in-service training in that it is also agency-based, and the agency is the primary beneficiary. But there is more emphasis on advancement of the individual professional and on the profession itself. Staff development tends to be broader in scope and concerned with more than just the rudimentary skills required of the task. Concern centers on developing staff capabilities and service delivery systems. Staff development is also more future-oriented than in-service training. The element of transferability is usually more extensive in staff development than with in-service training.

Continuing education, or professional development, is determined largely by the individual professional. It is more self-motivated than either in-service training or staff development. It may be self-directed. It can be long or short range in objectives. It can be broad or narrow in scope, depending on the learner's needs. The individual professional is the primary beneficiary (Council on Social Work Education, 1978).

Special Resource

One very good continuing education resource, developed during the past two years, is the Staff College, an intramural educational component of NIMH. The college provides a rich variety of educational offerings for community mental health center staff, including intensive seminars, experiential workshops, and back-home studies.

One of the persons responding to my survey on personnel and education highlights (1955-1980) was Richard Cravens (1980). About the Staff College and its importance for administrators, he wrote:

> There is a growing realization that a community mental health center is a business with an average budget of 2.0 M. Serving as an executive director of a CMHC requires special skills that are not developed by the traditional training found in the core disciplines. Consequently, training in administration for CMHC directors is recognized as necessary and training programs are becoming increas-

ingly available. *The NIMH staff college,* for example, offers training with respect to discrete subject matter designed to improved administrative capacity. In addition, a four-week intensive course is available touching in depth on a broad range of subject matter with the overall objective being to increase the managerial capacity of CMHC directors. Topics covered, for example, are labor negotiations, budgeting, decision making process, etc.

Growth

There has been impressive growth since 1955 in the design, volume, and quality of continuing education efforts. To illustrate the current range and volume, in social work alone, review of a Council on Social Work Education Report reveals that 25 universities alone offered over 350 workshops, institutes, seminars, and courses last summer. Prominent in the list were topics on abuse, rural services, rape, other forms of violence, and burnout (Continuing Education Programs, 1980).

Improvements in continuing education content and method have been greater, I believe, than in basic education where there is more "locking in" by tradition and where pressures for redesign are less. Campus audiences are more captive than continuing education ones. Postgraduate, on-the-job students are usually very discriminating and often highly critical. They have chosen the topic because of a felt need for improvement of work skills, not to gain credits for a degree. If the need is not met, the student in continuing education is usually quick to let the instructor know!

There are better linkages between continuing education and practice than exist between campus degree programs and practice. Continuing education in mental health also offers a broader sampling of models, such as medical, psychological-behavioral, social learning, social engineering, and combinations of these and others. Each of these models has validation and use, but overemphasis on one, or exclusion of others, creates education and service delivery problems. With so much that is still not known in our "fragile sciences," there is value in not getting locked into any one single approach. There are great opportunities for flexibility, diversity, and innovation in continuing education.

Example

From a wealth of continuing education projects during the past decade or two, many could be selected that are illustrative of progress during the period. I chose a recent, close-at-hand one, an NIMH-supported interdisciplinary project, Staff Board Collaboration in Community Mental Health Programs, 1975-79, which I directed.

Along with some successes, the project points up certain problems about continuing education design, methods, and content. I will extract some of these after briefly describing the project.

The project involved, on a voluntary basis, mental health professionals and board members affiliated with 24 Missouri community mental health centers, state hospitals, and their satellites. It was sponsored by the Social Work Extension Program, University of Missouri–Columbia, in cooperation with the Missouri Department of Mental Health.

The major purposes of the project were to:

(1) strengthen and enlarge board staff collaboration in design, development, interpretation, and funding of community mental health programs and services;
(2) extend the capacities of participating facilities for continuing education;
(3) develop teaching materials that would be useful to organizations involved in graduate and postgraduate education of mental health disciplines.

Following the successful conclusion of an earlier continuing education project (Ehrlich et al., 1970-73), and following careful assessment of continuing education needs with selected mental health facilities, the project and program were designed. They consisted of a series of workshops, seminars, and field practice experiences. Content included theory and practical application. Maximum utilization was made of self- and mutual education methods.

Three mental health centers in Kansas City participated in an intensive educational program consisting of a total of 83 seminars: 38 at one center, 26 at a second, and 19 at a third. In all, 45 board and staff members attended the seminars. Of these, about two-thirds were active on a sustained basis throughout the life of the project.

More limited educational experience was provided on a statewide basis for board and staff members from 21 additional centers, state hospitals, and their satellites. This consisted of two, two-day workshops spaced 1½ years apart. Combined workshop and seminar contact hours during the life of the project totaled almost 14,000.

The ratio of board to staff in seminars (Kansas City Area) was about 50-50. In workshops (statewide), board-to-staff ratio was about 40-60.

Major accomplishments included: strengthened staff-board educational collaboration in planning, programming, and services; development of replicable training models which can be adapted for use on a national, regional, statewide, or local basis; and production of a considerable range of education materials, including video cassettes.

Evaluation of the program's impact on individual, group, and organizational behavior and attitudes was an integrated part of the total project. Analysis of data, from questionnaires administered before and after the educational program, and from interviews with a sample of board and staff participants, indicated that the project impact, overall, was positive. The evaluators summarized: "The evidence indicates that the project had a favorable impact on the collaboration of board and staff, on overall functioning of board and staff, and on their attitudes toward community mental health."

Serendipitously, one year following the birth of the project idea in 1974, PL94-63 was passed by the National Congress. This legislation underlined and reinforced the importance of board/staff collaboration in design and operation of community mental health centers.

One of the basic assumptions of the project was that continuing education for staff and board members is essential if they are to work together effectively. A second assumption was that staff and board members should operate as peers in such an educational effort. Each has special expertise, experience, and problems to contribute.

A third assumption was that an adult education and participant leadership model is the best for such an educational effort, with maximum input of participants in the design and operation of a program. This model includes the use of experiences from the field on the part of both board and staff members.

Project experience confirmed these and other assumptions. A sample of quotes from board and staff participants succinctly sum up a few of the results:

(1) One board member, in conversation with one of the project research staff, spoke of increased understanding on her part about mental health and also increased self-esteem, importance, and assertiveness, as a board member, in her work with staff: "I got over sitting back. In one meeting, a psychiatrist kept talking about 'variegated treatment modalities.' After a while, I asked what that meant. I probed until the psychiatrist said, 'Patients are different and need different treatment.' I would never have questioned a psychiatrist before!"

(2) "We are making sure our board members are more than stamps of approval."

(3) "There is more of a sense of purpose or mission by the board and more recognition by the staff that the board can be helpful."

(4) "There was a lot of talk about collaboration, and we had to work out what it really meant for us. The collaboration issue was illustrated by the work on the program for the elderly. It involved how to work together, who had expertise, and where their skills were complementary."

(5) "The cost of the project was far outweighed by its benefits."

Problems

One persistent and troubling problem in the above project, particularly in the earlier stages, was with faculty/participant directed learning. It is not a problem unique to this project. It is one which continues in adult education efforts throughout the country.

The problem was well stated in a letter to me in 1974 from a friend and extension colleague, the late Professor Victor I.

Howery, Mental Health Continuing Education Program, University of Wisconsin. The letter followed Dr. Howery's review of an earlier continuing education project in Missouri on "Consultation in Community Mental Health Services."

In commenting about the project's mechanisms for engaging participants in their own learning direction, Dr. Howery wrote:

> In some of our work we have found it difficult to sustain groups over an extended period when we begin to expect the group and members of the group to assume a greater responsibility for inputs in the learning experience. *Adult learners create a real challenge for the programmer for adult learning.*
>
> If we accord a great deal of autonomy to *adult learners* and ask them to diagnose and design their own learning experiences, we get allegations that we are not assuming sufficient responsibility for content input. If *we* plan the structure and content, we face the accusation that we do not recognize their autonomy and individual needs and interests.
>
> As I read the material (consultation project report), I gained a greater sense for the mechanism you use in Missouri for engaging the members of the group and saw how you could meet some of the problems associated with a long-term learning experience.

In spite of considerable discussion (Staff Board Collaboration Project) and apparent agreement in the earlier stages with key staff and board members that the learning experience would be based on an adult education model, many project participants still anticipated a more traditional approach. There was a feeling on the part of some that they should be taught about the "hows" and "whys" of board/staff collaboration. The importance of their own contributions, both in the design and offering of educational content, was not fully accepted, and it was difficult to achieve a proper balance of didactic, theoretical, and experiential inputs.

Collaboration problems between project staff and participants, and board and staff members, also had wider significance in that they were related to the history of collaboration, or lack of it, in relation to many kinds of board/staff activities. Considerable work by the Project Coordinator on group climate building and maintenance was necessary. Essential, too, was assistance from him in balancing out some of the conflicting attitudes and values about group activities between the "take charge and let's get things done" approach with one of more collaborative agenda building, task formulation, and problem solving.

Some of these problems in self-directed learning are not unlike those I observe in university graduate seminars of various kinds of mental health and related professional students. They are so accustomed to being taught that they don't know how to behave in a seminar, or to appreciate the importance of their own contributions and the synergetic effects of sharing in group problem solving. This is a result of long conditioning in our educational system.

Some suggestions for these and other continuing education problems are offered in the final report of this project, along with details of other accomplishments and learning from the experience (Rieman et al., 1975-78).

CONCLUSION

Much research is needed regarding effective utilization and education of mental health professionals, both basic and continuing. Unfortunately, there has been a very serious decline in research funds during recent years for this purpose.

Even though additional research, theoretical and operational, is sorely needed, it seems to me that we have not made very effective use of what is already known. Much more is known than is applied. And distribution of research findings, as well as continuing education project experiences and reports, is sparse.

Funds for publication of project reports and evaluations are extremely limited. One is hard pressed to meet needs within one's own state, even though such findings have national value, too.

We still "reinvent the wheel" too many times in mental health programming, personnel utilization, and education. This is a luxury we can't afford, especially in these times of increasing service demands and declining budgets.

In concluding this panoramic sweep of progress during the past 25 years, I believe Cowper's words from "Winter Walk at Noon" speak for many of us in the fragile sciences:

> Knowledge is proud that he has learned so much.
> Wisdom is humble that he knows no more [Thatcher & McQueen, 1971: 108].

References

ADAMHA News. Economists to study MH system. February 1980, Volume *6*(4), 4. (a)

ADAMHA News. ADM facts heard at family conference. June 1980, *6*(12), 3. (b)

ADAMHA News. "Graduate" CMHC's seek renewed commitment. June 1980, *6*(12), 7. (c)

Continuing education programs in social work, spring and summer, 1980. Reported by graduate and undergraduate Social Work programs in colleges and universities, March 1980.

Council on Social Work Education. Notes on operational definitions of continuing social work education, staff development, in-service training and professional development. Unpublished manuscript, 1978.

CRAVENS, R. B. Letter to the author, June 24, 1980.

DAVENPORT, J. A., & DAVENPORT, J. III. *Boomtowns and human services.* Laramie: University of Wyoming, 1979.

DAVENPORT, J. A., & DAVENPORT, J. III. *The boom town: Problems and promises in the energy vortex.* Laramie: University of Wyoming, 1980.

EHRLICH, P. D., RIEMAN, D. W., & STRETCH, J. J. *Final report: Mental health and other community agency professionals–development, extension and utilization of mental health consultation, community organization and coordination skills and services.* Columbia: University of Missouri, 1970-1973.

GORDON, B. *I'm dancing as fast as I can.* New York: Harper & Row, 1979.

KATZ, A. A. *Encyclopedia of social work,* Vol. II. National Association of Social Workers, 1977.

KATZ, A. A., & BENDER, E. I. *The strength in us: Self-help groups in the modern world.* New York: Franklin Watts, 1976.

LEBEDUN, M., & SAMUELS, R. Staff productivity and program income in a CMHC. Paper presented at the annual meetings of the National Council of Community Mental Health Centers, San Francisco, February 20-23, 1980.

LOAVENBRUCK, G. Social work manpower research needs: Analysis in areas for future research. Unpublished manuscript, 1979.

MANNINO, F. V. *Mental health study center.* National Institute of Mental Health, 1969.

MANNINO, F. V., MacLENNAN, B. W., & SHORE, M. F. *Mental health study center.* National Institute of Mental Health, 1975.

National Broadcasting Corporation. *Six o'clock news,* June 23, 1980.

National Institute of Mental Health. *Community mental health center, the federal investment.* DHEW Publication No. (ADM) 78-677. Washington, DC: Government Printing Office, 1978.

The President's Commission on Mental Health. *Report to the President.* Washington, DC: Government Printing Office, 1978.

RAPOPORT, L. *National association of social workers,* 1963.

REIFF, R., & RIESSMAN, F. The indigenous nonprofessional. *Community Mental Health Journal,* 1965.

RIEMAN, D. W. *Mental health in the community public health program.* Austin: University of Texas, 1967.

RIEMAN, D., & McNEAL, J. *Prospectus: Community care service project for the mentally disabled.* Columbia: University of Missouri, 1980.

RIEMAN, D. W., CURRALL, J. F., Jr., BOWMAN, P. H., & NEFF, F. W. *Staff board collaboration in community mental health programs.* Columbia: University of Missouri, 1975-1978.

RUBIN, A. *Community mental health in the social work curriculum.* New York: Council on Social Work Education, 1979.

SANDALL, H. et al. The St. Louis community homes program: Graduated support for long-term care. *American Journal of Psychiatry,* June, 1975.

THATCHER, V. S., & McQUEEN, A. *The new Webster encyclopedic dictionary of the English language.* Chicago: Consolidated, 1971.

University of Missouri. *Field instruction manual, educational objectives.* Columbia: School of Social Work, 1978.

University of Missouri. *More than shelter–a play for reading.* Columbia: Extension Division, 1979. (a)

University of Missouri. UMC Social Work Extension Publication UED 41/300/1979. Columbia, 1979. (b)

VISCHI, T. R. et al. *The alcohol, drug abuse, and mental health national data book.* Washington, DC: Government Printing Office, 1980.

Part IV

ISSUES IN PRIMARY PREVENTION

Chapter 9

A CONCEPTUAL MODEL OF PREVENTION

PAUL V. LEMKAU

> He unfailingly attached his utopianism of consciousness to a psychological materialism: the absolute mind is also absolutely carnal.
>
> —Susan Sontag, 1980

The basis of the conceptual framework for the prevention of mental disorders presented in this chapter is that the fertilized ovum has represented in it the maxima of capacities the developed individual will ever be able to show. It follows from this that the prevention of mental, or indeed of all disorders of human behavior consists primarily of efforts to avoid the loss of capacities for behavior during the course of development from the fertilized ovum to the end of life.

Losses of capacities can occur through pathogenic events at any stage of development, from the earliest period to old age. Such events may include any of the known pathogenetic mechanisms, sociopsychological, traumatic, genetic, endocrinological, infectious, toxic, or nutritional. Illustrative examples of each of these are included below, and the second part of this chapter details examples of preventive programs, particularly relating to the sociopsychological area of pathogenesis.

PREVENTION AND THE MECHANISMS OF PATHOGENESIS

Disease and disorders are generally preventable only when the pathogenetic factor can be eliminated or when the mechanism by which the pathogenetic factor produces disease can be interfered with. A recent illustration of the elimination of a pathogenetic factor is found in the eradication of smallpox; there is, presumably, no longer any of the specific pathogen extant in the world except in rigorously monitored laboratories. An example of interference with the mechanism by which a pathogen produces disorder is found in the prevention of blindness in an unused strabismic eye by arranging that it share in seeing until it can be brought into continuous use, thus avoiding disuse atrophy. As amply illustrated in Eisenberg's (1981) review, both of these types of prevention apply in the prophylaxis of mental disorders. Eradication of smallpox eradicates smallpox and cowpox encephalitides with their dire behavior consequences. The same could be done with measles, syphilis, and other infectious processes that result in malfunction of the central nervous system.

The provision of appropriate stimulation for infants prevents the failure to thrive and grow as exemplified in such extreme cases as those presented by Spitz (1947) and in the marasmus described by Chapin (1908) in infants hospitalized in the pediatric hospitals of half a century ago. The recent demonstration of the reversibility of the suppression of the growth hormone in neglected and abused young children has opened new vistas for understanding and interfering with the pathogenetic mechanism in such cases (Money, 1977). Further illustrations in which similar interferences in patterns of child management in the perinatal, early childhood, and school developmental periods prevent the loss of inherent capacities or, conversely, promote their exhibition, are found mainly in the second part of this chapter. Much the same type of interference in the lifestyles of the elderly delays the behavioral effects of aging (Rodin, 1977).

A VIEW OF BEHAVIORAL PATHOLOGY

The pathology of behavior[1] may be of two types: (1) reduced capacity for and (2) reduced inhibition of behavior by changes in the functioning of the central nervous system. By far the commonest type of pathology is reduced function, be it the function of intelligence, as a symptom of mental retardation; apathy, as in some schizophrenic illnesses; or the amnesias of the elderly. Reduced inhibition of function is apparent in hallucinosis, delusion formation, and in elated and depressed moods. A convenient way of expressing these notions is that pathological behavior represents the amputation of part of the behavioral range or a tumorous growth upon it. "Amputation" and "tumors" of behavior occur in various combinations of "units" of behavior which are recognizable as syndromes and become named as mental or behavioral disorders. Mental retardation as a behavioral amputation is one which is reasonably measurable, so that the gradation of its presence can be observed and, to some degree, its extent correlated with the pathogenetic process or processes.

Other types of reduced range of behavior (adaptive disability in mental retardates and amnesias, for example) have not proved so easily quantifiable and remain largely as qualitative judgments. In spite of efforts to standardize and computerize the mental status examination, there is still not an H.Q. (hallucination quotient) or an A.Q. (apathy quotient) or a D.Q. (delusion quotient) with which to compare the behavior of one person with that of another. The evanescense of behavior "tumors" and their variation over time also contribute to the difficulties of measurement.

FACTORS INHERENT IN THE FERTILIZED OVUM WHICH DIMINISH CAPACITIES FOR BEHAVIOR

In some cases the fertilized ovum carries factors within its own chemical structure which penetrate during its development and cause behavioral disorders. It is known, for example, that spontaneously aborted fetuses show high rates of structural abnormalities; these and other types of deaths are included in the concept of "reproductive wastage" (Lilienfeld & Pasamanick, 1954), which includes the prenatal death of the individual and also the many interferences with growth and development as a kind of partial death—the loss of capacities necessary for full development.

Phenylketonuria is representative of the large group of disorders in which the fertilized ovum carries potentials for its own unhealthy development. It is one of the group—and the number is all too small to furnish great pride—in which the pathogenesis inherent in the fertilized ovum can be prevented, at least in many cases, from reducing the range of possible behavior, in this case through the restriction of intake of phenylalanine. Treatment not only allows the normal pigmentation of eyes and hair but also the normal or near-normal development of intelligence. The potential for mental deterioration inherent in the fertilized ovum is prevented from appearing in the individual by the management of a deviant metabolic process (Harper, 1962). The disorder has not been prevented, but the mechanism by which it produces pathological behavior has been interfered with, and the potential for a full range of behavior has been preserved.

A more common disorder inherent in the ovum is diabetes mellitus. The destructive potential inherent in the fertilized ovum can be thwarted by prompt diagnosis and substitutive treatment. Diabetes leads to arteriosclerosis, with its physical and mental symptomatology. Correcting the destructive potential of the fertilized ovum prevents the behavioral sequellae of the illness.

There are a large number of specific disorders inherent in the fertilized ovum which are not as yet preventable by metabolic management or substitutive therapy. Amniocentesis (USDHEW, 1979) makes possible the diagnosis of an increasing number of these, allowing a decision to be made as to whether the destructive potential should be allowed to mature so that an individual foredoomed to a limited existence—in time, or sociopsychologically—will be allowed to develop to delivery. Most would agree that embryos destined to the short and miserable life with Tay-Sachs disease ought not to be born. Similar judgments surround the prenatal diagnosis of incomplete closure of the neural canal (Gastell et al., 1980). Cases are not so easy to decide when the destructive potential is less catastrophic, as with Down's syndrome. It is wise to remember that when a fetus with inherent destructive potential is aborted, no disease has been prevented. What has been done is to make impossible the appearance of a case in the population.

Is there a possibility that genetic splicing might correct some of the destructive genetic potentials of the fertilized ovum? Perhaps, but certainly one should not be so rash as to hope for this at the present state of genetic engineering and in light of the tremendous emotional pressures in the area. However, the metabolic deficiency of human cells that produces Lesch-Nyham disease has been corrected in vitro using genetic material through E. Coli. This is a long way from preventing Lesch-Nyham disease, but it indicates a line of possible prevention for the future (Mulligan & Berg, 1980). It is conceivable that the pathogenetic process that leads to the "accident" resulting in Down's, which is (for one class of cases) more common in older mothers, may be discovered and corrected by manipulation of the environment within the mother. This is an end greatly to be desired and would relieve us of an ethical problem concerning the ultimate desirability of such individuals in the population.

Pathogenetic factors inherent in the fertilized ovum make themselves apparent in later periods of life than pre- and perinatally; witness Huntington's Chorea and, probably, at least some of the disorders of lipoid metabolism affecting myelin. Alzheimer's disease and arteriosclerosis are also probably, somehow and to some extent, controlled by factors inherent in the fertilized ovum (Kolata, 1981).

FACTORS WHICH MAY DIMINISH CAPACITY DURING THE INTRAUTERINE PERIODS OF DEVELOPMENT AND IN THE BIRTH PROCESS

The inherent potential of the fertilized ovum can be decreased by a number of pathogenic processes taking place in utero. Infection of the fetus when the mother contracts rubella is the best known example, and it has been demonstrated that the results of fetal rubella, deafness, cardiac defects, and mental retardation can be prevented by the immunization of prepubertal females (Harper, 1962). Fifty years ago, syphilis of the fetus was a matter of great concern; prompt diagnosis and treatment of the mother now prevents congenital syphilis, including its behavioral complications. Recently, the recognition of slow viruses as possible factors in the etiology of some behavior disorders has opened new avenues in the search for the prevention of diseases, including mental illnesses.

The recent recognition of the fetal alcohol syndrome has refocused attention on the effects of substances ingested by the mother in truncating the range of possible behaviors in the fetus (Jones & Smith, 1973). The thalidomide disaster of a decade ago demonstrated the responsibility of the medical and pharmacological sciences to obey the Hippocratian dictum: First do no harm. The "lead time" for the appearance of the effects of maternally ingested toxins can be very long; witness the effect of disylbesterol, used to control abortion in the mother, in reducing the ability of the female fetus to inhibit the appearance of vaginal carcinoma years later in her adolescence (USDHHS, 1981). One of the first of such decreases in the capacity of the fertilized ovum to be discovered was cretinism, the result of an insufficiency of iodine in the fetal environment (Rudolph, 1977).

Whether the psychological condition of the mother affects the maturation of the fetus she is carrying is moot. Traditionally, it was assumed that it did and in very direct ways. There is some evidence that a constantly anxious state in the mother tends to produce underweight and hyperactive infants at birth (Sontag & Richards, 1938). It has been demonstrated that emotionally disturbed mothers suffer more complications during pregnancy and at delivery than less disturbed mothers (Wooten, 1951). Cogan (1980) has reviewed material on the effect of prenatal education on delivery and the effectiveness of maternal care.

The effect of the mother's poor nutrition on the fetus is widely discussed as a factor that can reduce potential for development. The data are suggestive but not yet sufficiently clear to conclude that remedial programs are justifiable on this ground alone, attractive as they are for other reasons (Bergner & Susser, 1970).

Maternal vaginal bleeding during the third trimester of pregnancy has been etiologically associated with cerebral palsy. This association suggests that some such relationship could exist in the less catastrophic syndromes, such as "minimal brain damage" or hyperkenesis in children (Rutter, 1982). Preventive maneuvers are, however, as yet unclear for such conditions.

Obstetrical accidents may reduce inherent developmental capacity through direct trauma to tissue, anoxemia, or by hemorrhage. The preventive implications are so obvious that they will not be discussed further.

FACTORS REDUCING DEVELOPMENTAL CAPACITY OF THE FERTILIZED OVUM OCCURRING IN INFANCY AND EARLY CHILDHOOD

Developmental potential can be reduced in infancy and early childhood by many types of pathogenic factors, and various kinds of pathological processes may be involved.

Sociopsychological factors are clearly highly significant and have been understood for a long time. Homer Folks (Trattner, 1968) acted to replace orphanages with foster care before modern methods were available to document the scientific bases for his clinical conclusions. Chapin's (1908) successful efforts to prevent marasmus in hospitalized infants and Spitz's (1945) documentation of the failure of infants to develop in an unstimulating environment led to radical reforms based on mainly qualitative, clinical observation rather than quantitative, more specifically oriented clinical findings.

Bender (1947) supported these findings with data, and the field was reviewed by Bowlby (1951) in his book, *Maternal Care and Mental Health.* Modifications of Bowlby's original position have appeared, but the core concept of it remains valid, that infants deprived of language, and tactile and emotional contact with their caretakers do not thrive as well as those exposed to sufficient stimuli. Examples of preventive efforts in this area are included in Justice (Chapter 10, this volume).

Poisons, particularly lead, may destroy brain or peripheral nervous tissue and result in a reduction of the range of behavior or in the failure to inhibit pathological types of behavior (Casarett & Doull, 1975). Nutritional deprivation may have the same effect. The strategies for the prevention of such effects are very clear, though not all are equally effective in their application. Trauma to the brain, the largest proportion being secondary to inadequate restraints in auto accidents in this age group, is also responsible for the loss of inherent potential in the child (Baker, 1981).

FACTORS REDUCING DEVELOPMENTAL CAPACITY OF THE FERTILIZED OVUM IN CHILDHOOD AND ADOLESCENCE

The Headstart program in the United States represents a large-scale experiment to test the effect of a stimulating teaching environment in preparing young children to deal with the tasks presented by the educational system (Darlington et al., 1980). It appears that there are at least short-lived beneficial effects of such "nursery school" educational efforts to both the child and the parent, though the results of so widespread a program are very difficult to evaluate (Dill et al., 1975). Rutter et al. (1979) report a situation in which methods and organization of educational efforts later in the life of the child have been shown to improve the psychosocial functioning of the students involved.

FACTORS REDUCING DEVELOPMENTAL CAPACITY OF THE FERTILIZED OVUM IN ADULTHOOD

Child abuse and/or neglect are more prevalent among children of parents who have themselves been abused or neglected; it appears that their treatment as children somehow leads to failure to develop "normal" child-caring feelings and actions, a capacity presumed to have been environmentally thwarted. Justice (Chapter 10, this volume) reports on studies indicating the effectiveness of various ways of improving "mothering" which result in healthier children. There is little doubt that programs of preparation for pregnancy and childbirth are effective in increasing the proportion of births occurring with minimal anesthesia and fewer feelings of anxiety on the part of the mother, thus avoiding risks to the fetus (Cogan, 1980).

Epidemiological methods, as applied by Robbins (1973) in her studies of drug addiction in Vietnam veterans, have demonstrated the extent to which so profound an alteration of behavior (and neural substrate) as addiction can be changed through changed environmental circumstances.

Bereavement, particularly being widowed, is associated both with increased mortality and a higher prevalence of depressive disease in the surviving partner (Klerman & Izen, 1977), though the latter finding is less firm than the former, and Clayton (1974) disputes even that. The trauma of being widowed appears sufficient to cause the suppression of the individual's capacity to rebound after the loss. Kramer's (1976) work on the effect of available family on the admission and release from psychiatric (and other) hospitals deals not with the presence or absence of behavior disorder in the hospitalized patient but with a blockade by society of opportunities to exercise the capacity of the patient for living in the community.

Acute sensory deprivation produces pathologic behavior phenomena which can be relieved by restoration of the usual stimuli. A special case of sensory deprivation is, apparently, the intensive treatment wards of hospitals, where night and day are often indistinguishable and there are constant, repetitious sounds of monitors pervading and where, furthermore, the mechanics of existence take precedence over human interrelationships. The restructuring of the way of life on these wards appears to have reduced the incidence of deleria occurring in this setting (Weiss, 1976).

The use of drugs, particularly LSD (Paulsen, 1970) and marijuana (Szymanski, 1981), appears in some cases to reduce the capacity of the individual to inhibit pathological behaviors once the pattern of reaction has been established. Prevention of such drug-induced facilitation reactions (flashback) at present appears to be a matter of the avoidance of the original use of consciousness-altering drugs.

Leighton et al. (1963) show that broader societal factors may reduce the potential of individuals within a social group to avoid certain symptoms, mostly of the syndromes usually considered "neurotic" or "psychosomatic."

Three communities, one rather highly organized along Protestant religious and social ideals, including active participation in community functions by women, one organized under the strong influence of the Catholic church, and one in which no predominant organizing force was apparent, were surveyed. The community lacking a predominant culture (unorganized) produced a larger proportion of symptomatic individuals than did the other two. No evidence was submitted to indicate that efforts to "organize" an unorganized community would reduce the proportion of symptomatic people, however.

De Figuereido (1975) has shown that members of the Goan population who were subject to the greatest stresses of adaptation in that population of mixed, predominantly Portuguese and predominantly native cultures had the greatest proportion of symptomatic people in its members.

Looked at from the point of view of massive population aggregates, persons whose lives are "out of fit" with the population norms show larger proportions of mentally disordered individuals than those falling within the norms (Wechsler & Pugh, 1967). Thus, the divorced, never-married, and widowed in the population show more symptoms and gross mental disease than those who marry and stay married. In none of the instances mentioned has it been demonstrated that alteration of the social system or the individual's place in it will change the prevalence of symptoms in the population.

The pathogenic process is not understood, and no clear preventive strategy is presently apparent. Epidemiological studies generally also support the thesis that symptoms appear in higher prevalence in the poverty-stricken than in the better-off segments of the population. Although the "chicken or the egg" dilemma also appears in this case, many governments have instituted social welfare programs with the purpose of relieving the obvious stresses that play on the deprived groups. There is as yet no evidence that these programs actually reduce symptomatology in the recipients of such welfare services; the pathogenicity of cultural and financial poverty and the efficacy of the purportedly preventive efforts remain untested.

FACTORS REDUCING CAPACITY IN OLDER AGE GROUPS

Progress has been made in the specification of the organ and cellular pathology occurring in cases of senile psychosis, and again, there is evidence that the pathogenetic potential lies in the fertilized ovum—a heritable factor of very late expression (Kolata, 1981). No predictive markers are known.

The process of aging pervades the whole of the individual; the heart has less reserve, and the same is true of the lungs, the kidney, the brain, and the skeleton. In all probability, the maintenance or increase of function of any organ or system of organs would serve to stave off the psychological symptoms of senility or other mental disorder in the aged. Aging and senility are general medical problems which mental health specialists share with all their colleagues in the helping professions.

There appear to be some pathogenetic factors of sociopsychological origin that result in an overly rapid decrease in behavioral potential in the elderly. For the most part, these relate to the concept that without the stimulative use of capacities, the range of potential behaviors becomes narrowed. It is assumed that if sociopsychological behaviors are not "exercised," they will disappear more rapidly than otherwise; the homology is to "disuse atrophy." This process can be interfered with through efforts to preserve social, language, and problem-solving skills for as long as possible.

Thinking along these lines is not new. Martin and De Gruchy published a highly stimulating book on the subject as early as 1930, although no quantitative material was presented. Rodin (1977) tested the hypothesis that persons living in nursing homes would be healthier if they were given greater responsibility and control over their activities. She showed that a test group given more opportunities to control their activities and followed for three years lived longer, had less illness, and felt healthier than a comparison group who were not encouraged to be self-directing.

SUMMARY

The conceptual framework for the prevention of mental disorders presented in this section is that prophylactic efforts are to be aimed at preserving the full range of behavioral functions inherent in the fertilized ovum, and in preventing the exhibition of any potentials for inadequate behavior that may be inherent in the fertilized ovum.

Prophylaxis may be a matter of interfering with pathogenetic processes, as in the prevention of rubella in pregnant women by early immunization; of controlling a pathogenetic metabolic function, as in phenylketonuria; of supplying necessary nutrients, as in cretinism; or of providing psychosocial experiences essential to optimum development, as through teaching "mothering" to infant caretakers, providing stimulating cultural and educational opportunities to young children, well planned and monitored educational experiences to youngsters, adequate psychosocial stimulation to adults, and stimulating experiences to aging persons. The prevention of mental disorders includes avoidance of substances which directly poison and kill brain tissue, as well as substances that poison and/or leave traces that facilitate malfunction, as in the nature of flashbacks.

The obverse of this concept is that mental health may be promoted more or less irrespective of the inherent capacities of the individual concerned. This is a highly attractive idea allowing great optimism for the amelioration of the human condition. Its danger lies in that it allows the raising of unfounded hopes, followed by disappointment and disillusion. Furthermore, it seems to this writer to spawn fads in the management of personality development which, requiring no scientific basis, lead to crashes of public confidence in the more plodding, less gaudy methods that can be formulated as hypotheses, put into experimental operation, and tested for effectiveness.

AN ADDED NOTE ON THE PREVENTION OF SCHIZOPHRENIA AND AFFECTIVE PSYCHOSES

These two diseases and their clinical variations constitute the major therapeutic and prophylactic challenges to the mental health professions. Neither is discussed in this chapter because neither the etiology nor the mechanisms by which these diseases are produced are clear. In both, the last decades have seen enormous growth in the neurophysiology of the diseases and equally in methods of therapy or control of symptoms.

It is probably the fact that no means is known of controlling the incidence of these groups of illnesses which has led to such great recurrent waves of disillusionment concerning the preventability of "mental disease." It must be kept in mind that there is no "mental disease"; there are a great many mental diseases. Some are clearly preventable, some no one knows how to prevent. It appears wise, when one is considering prevention, to clearly formulate which disease, disorder, or syndrome one's effort is directed at preventing. Perhaps care in the stating of aims will smooth the course of progress toward the prevention of an ever-larger proportion of mental disorders, making it smoother and less marked by overenthusiasm and subsequent disillusionment.

NOTE

1. "Behavior" is defined here, as by Adolf Meyer, to include thinking and feeling.

REFERENCES

BAKER, S. Private Communication, 1981.

BENDER, L. Psychopathic behavior disorders in children. In R. M. Lindner and R. V. Seliger (Eds.), *Handbook of correctional psychiatry.* New York, 1947.

BERGNER, L., & SUSSER, M. W. Low birth weight and prenatal nutrition: An interpretative review. *Pediatrics,* 1970, *46,* 946.

BOWLBY, J. *Maternal care and mental health.* Geneva: World Health Organization, 1951.

CASARETT, L. J., & DOULL, J. *Toxicology.* New York: Macmillan, 1975.

CHAPIN, H. D. A plan of dealing with atrophic infants and children. *Archives of Pediatrics,* 1908, *25,* 491-496.

CLAYTON, P. Mortality and morbidity in the first year of widowhood. *Archives of General Psychiatry,* 1974, *25,* 745-750.

COGAN, R. Effects of childbirth preparation. *Obstetrics & Gynecology,* 1980, *23,* 1-14.

DARLINGTON et al. Preschool programs and later school competence of children from low income families. *Science,* 1980, *208,* 202-204.

DILL, J. R. et al. Comparative indices of school achievements by black children from different preschool programs. *Psychological Reports,* 1975, 871-877.

EISENBERG, L. A research framework for evaluating the promotion of mental health and prevention of mental illness. *Public Health Reports,* 1981, *96,* 3-19.

DE FIGUEREIDO, J. M. Change and disintegration: An investigation in cultural psychiatry. Thesis, The Johns Hopkins School of Hygiene and Public Health, 1975.

GASTELL, B. et al. (Eds.) *Maternal serum alpha-feto protein: Issues in the prenatal screening and diagnosis of neural tube defects.* Washington DC: Government Printing Office, 1980.

HARPER, P. A. *Preventive pediatrics.* New York: Appleton-Century-Crofts, 1962.

JONES, K. L., & Smith, D. W. Fetal alcohol syndrome. *Lancet,* 1973, *2,* 999-1001.

KLERMAN, G. L., & IZEN, J. E. The effects of bereavement and grief on physical health and general well-being. Adv. Psycho. Med. 1977, *9,* 63-104.

KOLATA, G. M. Clues to the cause of senile dementia. *Science,* 1981, *211,* 1032-1033.

KRAMER, M. Issues in the development of statistical and epidemiological data for mental health services research. *Psychological Medicine,* 1976, *6,* 185-215.

LEIGHTON, D. et al. *The character of danger.* New York: Basic Books, 1963.

LILIENFELD, A., & PASAMANICK, B. The association of maternal and foetal factors with the development of epilepsy, I: Abnormalities in the prenatal and perinatal periods. *Journal of the American Medical Association,* 1954, *155,* 719-724.

MARTIN, L. J., & DeGRUCHY, C. *Salvaging old age.* New York: Macmillan, 1930.

MONEY, J. The syndrome of abuse dwarfism (psychosocial dwarfism or reversible hyposomatotropism). American Journal of Disabled Children, 1977, *131,* 508-513.

MULLIGAN, R. C., & BERG, P. Expression of a bacterial gene in mammalian cells. *Science,* 1980, *209,* 1422-1427.

PAULSEN, J. Psychiatric problems. In R. H. Blum and Associates (Eds.), *Students and drugs II: College and high school observations.* San Francisco: Jossey-Bass, 1970.

ROBBINS, L. N. *The Vietnam drug user returns.* Washington, DC: Government Printing Office, 1973.

RODIN, J. Long-term effects of a control-relevant intervention with the institutionalized aged. *Journal of Personality and Social Psychology,* 1977, *35,* 897-902.

RUDOLPH, A. M. (Ed.) *Pediatrics.* New York: Appleton-Century-Crofts, 1977.

RUTTER, M. Syndromes attributed to minimal brain dysfunction in childhood. American Journal of Psychiatry, 1982, *139,* 21-33.

RUTTER, M. et al: Fifteen Thousand Hours: Secondary Schools and Their Effects on Children. Cambridge, Mass., Harvard U. Press, 1979.

SONTAG, L. W., & RICHARDS, T. W. *Fetal heart rate as a behavior indicator.* Washington, DC: National Research Council, 1938.

SONTAG, S. *Under the sign of Saturn.* New York: Farrar, Straus, Geroux, 1980.

SPITZ, R. Emotional growth in the first year. *Child Study,* 1947, *24,* 68-70.

SZYMANSKI, H. V. Prolonged depersonalization after marijuana use. American Journal of Psychiatry, 1981, *138,* 231-233.

TRATTNER, W. I. *Homer Folks: Pioneer in social welfare.* New York: Columbia University Press, 1968.

U.S. Department of Health, Education and Welfare. Antenatal diagnosis. Washington, DC: Public Health Service, 1979.

U.S. Department of Health and Human Services. Prenatal diethylstilbesterol (DES) exposure: Recommendation of the diethylstilbesterol-adenosis (DESAD). NIH Publication No. 81-2049. Washington, DC: Government Printing Office.

WECHSLER, H., & PUGH, T. C. Fit of individual and community characteristics and rates of psychiatric hospitalization. American Journal of Sociology, 1967, *731,* 331-338.

WEISS, H. J. Psychological aspects of intensive care. In J. L. Berk et al., *Handbook of critical care.* Boston: Little, Brown, 1976.

WOOTEN, B. G. The emotional status of 56 prenatal clinic patients: Correlation with obstetrical experience. Thesis, The Johns Hopkins School of Hygiene and Public Health, 1951.

Chapter 10

PRIMARY PREVENTION
Fact or Fantasy?

BLAIR JUSTICE

The debate over whether primary prevention in the mental health field is fact or fantasy seems to center on two questions: (1) With our present state of knowledge, what can we prevent? and (2) What, if any, demonstrable effects can we point to as evidence of success? This is not to say that there are not other issues of controversy, such as the expense involved and the training of those who may carry out preventive activities. But these two areas—what we can prevent and how we know that our efforts are effective—are at the core of the question: Is primary prevention in the mental health field fact, or is it fantasy?

The first issue that must be dealt with is: What can we prevent? Hollister (1977) notes that humility is the keynote in setting the goals of prevention programs. Until the day when we learn how to prevent the major psychoses and character disorders, we must settle for more limited objectives. Until the day when we can prevent such major disorders as schizophrenia, it is helpful to remember (as Hollister notes) that even in physical

Author's Note: I wish to acknowledge the assistance on this chapter of Pam Lewis, Ph.D. candidate in behavioral sciences at the University of Texas School of Public Health.

medicine, the first preventive efforts were not to prevent serious disease processes such as heart disease, cancer, or arthritis, but rather to prevent injuries, hemorrhages, wound infection, and the like.

Toward the end of this chapter, I will cite activities in several states where programs are underway and prevention efforts, at least, are very much a fact, not a fantasy. These represent a real beginning.

WHAT IS A MENTAL HEALTH PROBLEM?

Those who believe that primary prevention of mental disorders is fantasy cite the "fuzziness of concepts and definitions underlying the issues." Most recently, Lamb and Zusman (1979) have taken this position. They note that "unless care is taken to distinguish prevention of diagnosable mental illness from prevention of unhappiness, feelings of distress, or social incompetence, discussants will often be examining several different phenomena while thinking they are focusing on one." The assumption basic to most primary prevention programs, according to Lamb and Zusman, is that difficult life circumstances lead to mental illness, and this assumption is as yet unproved. The major problem with this argument is that Lamb and Zusman (and many others opposed to primary prevention in the mental health area) do not give us a definition of diagnosable mental illness. Is it only those conditions where actual brain disease can be demonstrated or histopathology detected? There are countless more mental health problems that produce distress and dysfunction that do not seem to have a biological defect as the central issue. To suggest that these are minor problems, or that they should not be our area of concern, is to discount the extreme importance of psychosocial factors and the damaging effect they can have on millions of lives.

To make clear what I am considering a mental health problem, I am borrowing the pragmatic approach of Munoz (1976) and defining primary prevention this way: It is any effort that reduces "the probability of occurrence of those problems which are presently referred to mental health personnel." These problems may or may not fit discrete diagnostic categories, but generally involve difficulties in thought, perceptions, feelings, and/or behavior (Munoz & Kelley, 1975). In this vein, Hollister (1977) has proposed some direct goals of prevention, including common problems presently referred to mental health personnel, such as specific self-defeating behaviors, role failures, relationship breakdowns, emotional overreactions, and other psychological disturbances.

STRESS MODEL

As suggested by the Task Panel on Prevention of the President's Commission on Mental Health (1978: 1847), a stress model is needed to provide us with the means to conceptualize the mental health problems for which we want to design primary prevention strategies. Stress may be defined as the internal response we experience when subjected to stimuli that threaten our survival or emotional needs. We call these stimuli "stressors."

Hollister (1979) states that the four major strategies of primary prevention are: (1) stressor management, where the focus is on managing the stimuli before they have an impact on the person; (2) stressor avoidance, where it is possible to get some of the vulnerable persons away from feeling the impact of specific stimuli; (3) stress resistance building, that is, mobilizing strength-building experiences that will enable persons in the target group to resist more readily the effects of stress; and (4) stress reaction management, which overlaps with secondary prevention and prevents progression of a disturbance once the person has already felt the impact of stress. This, then, is the model from which we will examine specific prevention efforts.

We will see that the first question about whether primary prevention is fact or fantasy may be answered as follows: It is fact if the goals are modest and specific and are directed toward problems currently referred to mental health personnel. It is fantasy if goals are global and nonspecific—for example, to prevent "mental illness," major psychoses, or to make sweeping, societal changes.

The second question to be addressed is: What, if any, are demonstrable prevention effects? If we are to know for certain that our efforts are effective, we must use rigorous evaluation as a matter of course in our program design. The use of control groups that do not receive intervention is essential to give us an idea of the expected rate of change in the outcome variables. These outcome variables must also be quantifiable if we are going to be able to talk about relative magnitudes of change. We need to be able to say how much of an effect the program had and to specify the mediating cognitive and behavioral skills involved. As we have said, limited, specifiable goals are easier to evaluate than more global ones, and only through this approach can we presently hope to show that it is possible to produce preventive effects. Clear interpretation of the findings and their practical significance is also necessary. Aside from the question of effect (Did the program work?), evaluation must also deal with cost effectiveness (Was this the least costly method that could produce the desired effect?).

QUANTIFIABLE VARIABLES

After looking at some examples of primary prevention programs, we will see that the second question as to whether primary prevention is fact or fantasy may be answered as follows: It is fact if variables are specifiable in quantitative terms and if it is shown that the intervention program is the most probable cause of the change observed. It is fantasy if we cannot talk about relative magnitudes of change or if findings are not of practical significance.

The characteristics, then, of primary prevention programs of fact, as opposed to fantasy, can be summed up as follows:

(1) The programs should address high-risk families or groups as opposed to individuals with already observed pathology.
(2) They should use control groups.
(3) They should use quantifiable dependent variables.
(4) They should specify mediating cognitive and behavioral skills that may be evaluated as intermediate goals.

The characteristics of primary prevention programs of fantasy, or programs of questionable value, include the following:

(1) They try to make major societal or organizational changes.

(2) They lack rigorous research design and do not include control groups.

Now let us examine specific primary prevention programs as they relate to the stress model strategies mentioned earlier. Each of the programs examined here will meet the criteria of "primary prevention programs of fact." That is, each will have specific, limited goals aimed toward problems which may be referred to mental health personnel, and each will use specifiable, quantifiable variables and a control group. All will use one of the four stress model strategies: stressor management, stressor avoidance, stress resistance building, and stress reaction management. We will explore at least one example of primary prevention programming for each strategy. These programs cover a wide range of ages (from infants through widows) and a wide range of problems (the prevention of school dropouts, complications of surgery, and maladjustment in children).

PREVENTION BY MODIFYING STRESSORS

First let us look at *stressor management interventions.* These are programs designed to decrease or modify some or all of the stressors that might create disturbances in specific target groups. The example here concerns the work of Dr. Elsie Broussard (1977). She designed the Neonatal Perception Inventory (NPI), which uses the mother's concept of the average baby as the basis for comparing her own infant's behavior. The Pittsburgh First-Born Preventive Intervention Program was designed to provide intervention for high-risk infants as identified by the NPI. Such infants were judged to be at high risk of future emotional disorders. This project included 281 healthy, first-born infants who were, on the basis of the NPI, placed in a low-risk group (205) or a high-risk group (76). Using a random method, the high-risk group was divided into 39 to whom intervention was offered and 37 to whom no intervention was offered. The program consisted of supplementary parenting through weekly mother-infant group meetings plus home visitation. One goal was to give the mother a new image of a potential relationship through the staff's parenting of the mother. It was expected that as the mother herself felt valued and respected and her child valued and respected, she would begin to modify her self-perception and her perception of the child.

At one year of age, 84 of the infants were evaluated: 34 low-risk and 60 high-risk (16 Intervention, 14 Intervention-Refused, and 20 Comparison subjects). A statistically significant difference ($p < .05$) was evident between high- and low-risk infants, with the low-risk having more optimal scores on four clinical clusters related to emotional disturbance. Within the high-risk group, the comparison group had the more deviant scores. Scores were not significantly different, but the trend was in the expected direction: Although disturbance at age 1 had not been totally prevented, the mean scores of the intervention group were closer to the low-risk group than were the comparison group to whom no intervention had been offered.

AVOIDING HARMFUL IMPACT

The next strategy is *stressor avoidance intervention.* This strategy is based on keeping vulnerable persons from experiencing the impact of harmful stressors, that is, to arrange to withdraw them from potentially disabling situations or encounters.

The example here is from the work of Kennel et al. (1976) on parent-infant bonding. They note that mothers separated from their babies during the first hours after delivery often have difficulty forming an attachment to their infants, and that this can later play a part in potential child abuse. Thus, the stressor to be avoided in this case is the separation of mother and infant. A total of 14 mothers who made up the "early and extended contact" group in this study were given routine contact with their babies and were also given their nude babies in bed for one hour in the first two hours after delivery and for five extra hours on each of the next three days of life. The control group of 14 mothers received the care that is routine in most U.S. hospitals.

The mothers returned to the hospital 28-32 days after delivery for three separate observations to determine if the additional mother-infant contact had resulted in altered maternal behavior. The authors report significant differences between the two groups in all three observations. Mothers who had extended early contact with their babies were found to pick their babies up more, look at them more, talk to them more, and spend more time with them. This pattern was still found to be present two years later.

RESISTING EFFECTS OF STRESS

The third strategy is *stress resistance building.* The effort here is to mobilize strength-building experiences that will enable persons in the target group to resist more readily the effects of stress. Anticipatory guidance is a type of stress-resistance strategy involving timing a specific preparatory strength-building intervention to occur just before exposure to an anticipated crisis. There are a number of prevention program examples that demonstrate this popular strategy.

The first one concerns the work of Skipper and Leonard (1968). Their study dealt with some of the effects of hospitalization and surgery—physiological, as well as social and psychological—in young children. Much of children's behavior while hospitalized for surgery is presumed to be a response to psychological and physiological stress. This experiment was designed to test the effects on the behavior of hospitalized children of a nurse's interactions with the children's mothers. The hope was that the experiment would develop a method of reducing the children's stress indirectly by reducing the stress of their mothers. An important means of reducing stress from potentially threatening events is through the communication of information about the event. In all, 80 patients were randomly assigned to experimental and control conditions (40 to each). These conditions consisted of regular admission procedures and nursing care. Experimental conditions began when the mother and child went through admission procedures at the hospital. Although the child was present, the focus of interaction was the mother. The special nurse attempted to create an atmosphere that would facilitate the communication of information to the mother, maximize freedom to verbalize her fear and anxiety and to ask all the questions that were on her mind. The authors note that "information given to the mother tried to paint an accurate picture of the reality of the situation–what routine events to expect and when they were likely to occur including the actual time schedule for the operation" (Skipper & Leonard, 1968). This procedure took about five minutes longer than regular admission procedures. The special nurse also met with experimental mothers for about five minutes at several other times before and after the operation.

Somatic measures of the children's stress were recorded at admission, preoperatively, postoperatively, and at discharge. These consisted of temperature, systolic blood pressure, and pulse rate. Eight days after discharge, mothers were mailed questionnaires concerning the hospital experience and its aftermath. Nursing staff also completed independent measures of each mother's level of stress and general adaptation to the hospital.

Findings included the following: Results of the mail-back questionnaire revealed that experimental group mothers suffered less stress than control group mothers during and after the operation. This finding was substantiated by the independent evaluation of the regular nursing staff. Also, differences in temperature, blood pressure, and pulse rate between experimental and control children were apparent, especially at discharge. With regard to blood pressure and pulse rate, the differences were statistically significant (beyond the .005 level). Results of the mail-back questionnaire also revealed that the experimental group children seemed to experience fewer physiological ill effects from the operation and made a more rapid recovery than control group children. There were also major social and psychological behavioral differences between the groups in three areas: excessive crying, disturbed sleep, and an unusual fear of doctors, nurses, and hospitals (these differences also reached levels of statistical significance). Skipper and Leonard concluded that a change in the quality of interaction between an authoritative person, such as the experimental nurse, and the hospitalized child's mother can ultimately result in less stress for the child and consequently a change in his social, psychological, and even physiological behavior.

The work of Skipper and Leonard, as well as the work of Broussard, which we reviewed previously, points to the importance of social support as a moderator of life stress. Cobb (1976) conceives of social support as information belonging to one or more of the following three classes:

(1) information leading the subject to believe that he is cared for and loved;
(2) information leading the subject to believe that he is esteemed and valued; and
(3) information leading the subject to believe that he belongs to a network of communication and mutual obligation.

Results of the Skipper and Leonard study support Cobb's concept of social support as protection against the development of both physiological and psychological reactions to stress.

Broussard's use of supplementary parenting through mother-infant groups also illustrates the importance of social support. As we saw, one goal of these groups was to help the mothers feel valued and respected so that they could begin to modify their self-perceptions and their perceptions of their children.

COPING SKILLS

The next example of the stress-resistance-building strategy is the prevention work of Spivack and Shure (1977). Their study focuses on increasing coping skills among low-income children to prevent behavioral problems. Their early research indicates that "individuals deficient in interpersonal problem solving skills are significantly more poorly adjusted than those more efficient in such skills." As a result, their programs have emphasized teaching nursery and kindergarten children various alternatives to typical problematic situations in their lives and to consider potential consequences of interpersonal acts. They put together building blocks judged necessary for efficient interpersonal problem-solving. These included listening, language skills, rudiments of logic, the concept of multiple attributes, fairness and consequences, the labeling of human emotions, and the incorporation of all these skills into actual problem solving. The specific objective of their Philadelphia project was to evaluate the effect of interpersonal problem-solving skills on behavioral adjustment.

Results included the following: The position was supported that interpersonal problem-solving skills function as a direct mediator of behavioral adjustment. The skills most affected were alternative and consequential thinking. Compared with nontrained controls, one year of training was sufficient to improve behavior. Training effects lasted at least two full years after training. A preventive effect of the program was also indicated: Significantly more trained than nontrained youngsters who were normally adjusted throughout the nursery year maintained that adjustment throughout kindergarten and first grade. Adjustment was judged by the child's teacher each year.

ENRICHING IQ IN CHILDREN

The third example of stress resistance building is the Milwaukee Project. This project began before the birth of its subjects. A survey of a low-income neighborhood in Milwaukee found that low maternal intelligence scores were the best single predictor of low intelligence scores in children. The type of retardation being investigated was "cultural familial mental retardation," a condition without identifiable gross pathology of the central nervous system found almost exclusively among the economically depressed. The project selected 40 low-income mothers whose full-scale WAIS Score was less than 75 and who had just given birth. The sample was restricted to black families to reduce cultural and racial variability. Of the newborns, 20 were assigned to a control condition and 20 to the preventive program.

Babies began the program between 3 and 6 months of age and continued it until they entered first grade. The program lasted all day, five days per week, 12 months per year. The focus was on perceptual/motor skills, cognitive/language development, and social/emotional growth in the babies. All but one of the teachers were paraprofessionals, and the program was located in the families' neighborhoods.

A second focus was on the mothers. A rehabilitation program was designed to prepare them for employment opportunities, as well as to improve their homemaking and childrearing skills. Results of the study to date are as follows: (1) Standard intelligence tests, in which both groups started at comparable levels, began to diverge at about 18 months of age. By 66 months of age, the experimental groups obtained a mean IQ of 122 while the controls obtained a mean of 91. (2) Learning measures also showed better results for the experimental group. (3) Language measures favored the experimental children, who said more than controls and had larger vocabularies. (4) Social and personality measures also favored the experimentals, in that they guided interpersonal interactions more, and questioned as well as taught their mothers during task performance situations.

The control group is now starting to show a decline in IQ scores—an often observed phenomenon in "cultural-familial retarded." The experimental group has not followed suit.

The Philadelphia Project and the Milwaukee Project point to the importance of competence training in a stress-resistance strategy of prevention. The Prevention Task Panel of the President's Commission on Mental Health (1978) notes that the competency training model has been shown to be useful across diverse settings and age, sex, ethnic, and socioeconomic levels, as indicated in the two examples just discussed. The task panel has stated:

> We now know that several pivotal competencies, on the surface quite far removed from mental health's classic terrain, can be taught effectively to young children and that their acquisition radiates positively to adaptations and behaviors that are, indeed, of prime concern to mental health. Symptoms and problem behaviors are reduced after acquisition of these skills. Health has been proactively engineered, so to speak, through skill acquisition. This is a message we cannot afford to repress; it is both a paradigmatic example and further mandate for intensified primary prevention efforts.

REDUCING VULNERABILITY

Although our review of examples to this point has focused on prevention programs involving children and young infants, there are also examples of programs that focus on adults of all ages. Within the stress resistance building strategy, for example, is Bloom's (1971) work with 200 freshman college students. The unusual vulnerability of college freshmen to stresses during the early months of college is well known. Bloom notes that "while about 5% of the student body in the average university seeks psychiatric help each year, the incidence of help-seeking is unusually high among freshmen. The drop-out rate is twice as high for freshmen as for seniors and it has been suggested that freshmen constitute a specific high-risk group due to the difficulties of the role transition associated with living away from home as a college student."

Among other things, Bloom's project was designed to (1) provide a sense of membership in a group and thus reduce feelings of isolation; (2) provide group members with some tools by which to understand better the stresses acting on them and their reactions to these stresses; and (3) provide a resource person for the students to talk with in the event of some crisis. The intervention was primarily an ongoing process between these students and the investigator around issues of crisis and adjustment which the students were experiencing. Students were followed regardless of whether they remained on the campus or went elsewhere.

Evaluations of the pilot project were generally favorable. In contrast to a comparison group of freshmen, the experimental group had a somewhat higher survival rate, and of those no longer on the campus, a significantly larger portion of experimental group students continued their academic involvement in other settings. In addition, of students who left the university, a majority of the members of the experimental group continued to live away from home, while a majority of the comparison groups returned to their parents' home. The favorable results from Bloom's pilot project may be due to a combination of its social support aspects (membership in the project) and its competency-building aspect (giving students the tools by which to understand the stresses acting on them, as well as their reactions).

RELIEVING GRIEF REACTIONS

Let us now consider the final strategy for prevention programs—*stress reaction management.* The effort here is to prevent the person's response to stressors from compounding his problems—that is, to prevent progression of a problem once the person has already felt the impact of stress. This strategy actually overlaps with secondary prevention, as Hollister (1977) notes. In both examples here, the focus is on social support networks for persons in crisis. To date, neither of these two programs has reported quantified outcome measures or the use of a control or comparison group—thus, neither strictly meets our criteria for primary prevention programs of "fact." Both, however, are generally recognized as being of potential value and importance.

The first example is the work of Silverman (1972). She found that newly widowed persons rarely consider using traditional mental health-related agencies unless they had utilized them prior to widowhood. Rather, what is more appropriate is a service that is available immediately after a death occurs that can reach every new widow and that can provide a range of services, including all existing community services. This ongoing program is designed to facilitate the transition from role of wife to role of widow in newly widowed persons under 65 years of age. The method employed utilizes as helping agents other widows who have themselves successfully made the transition. Silverman notes that the findings of the Widow-to-Widow program indicate that widows and widowers often develop emotional disturbance when they cannot give up their role of wife or husband—that is, when they continue to live as they had when their spouse was alive. The widow aides must help the new widow give up the role of wife, return to earlier roles (such as paid worker), or establish new roles, deal with the secondary mourning that often emerges six months or a year after the spouse's death, and resume a socializing lifestyle. The widow aide can talk about her own grief and become a role model and a bridge back to the real world.

In the first 1 1/2 years of the program, efforts were made to reach 300 newly widowed persons. Of the 233 who were reached, 61 percent accepted at least some of the widow-aide services. Younger widows (especially those with children and those who were not working) were most receptive. The problems discussed included housing, childrearing, finances, difficulties with relatives, and job training. Widows needed assurance that they could successfully weather the difficulties they faced, and talking with someone who had coped with the same problem was clearly beneficial.

The second example of a stress reaction management strategy is Goldston's work (1977), which concerns itself with the mental health needs in families experiencing Sudden Infant Death Syndrome (SIDS). Between 7,500 and 10,000 babies die annually from SIDS. Surviving parents and siblings are often characterized by a pervasive grief and guilt reaction that may result in severe family dysfunction, divorce, and disability. Like the widows mentioned earlier, most bereaved families will not reach out for help from either a mental health facility or private practitioner. Mutual help groups composed of parents of SIDS victims have been found to be effective mental health resources for newly bereaved families. In addition to the mutual help groups, Goldston also advocates and works to implement public education projects to promote greater awareness about the characteristics of normal grief reactions, as well as some of the harmful cultural myths relating to comforting the bereaved ("Don't think about the past"; "Get pregnant as soon as possible," and so forth).

BARRIERS TO PREVENTION EFFORTS

This review of programs and interventions illustrates that primary prevention activities can have an impact. Although it is a fact that primary prevention is possible and there are programs with demonstrable results, primary prevention on a large scale may remain a fantasy unless certain obstacles are overcome. These include:

(1) the lack of funding for primary prevention and the "catch-22" demand that funds should not be made available until results are demonstrated;

(2) the lack of any organization whose primary job is to implement and coordinate primary prevention;
(3) the lack of any cadre of professionals trained specifically to develop, carry out, and evaluate primary prevention programs.

The Task Panel on Prevention of the President's Commission on Mental Health (1978) notes two other points that serve as barriers to primary prevention efforts: (1) Our society is crisis-oriented while primary prevention is future-oriented and thus postponable; and (2) The history, traditions, and past values of the mental health professions have been built on treating existing dysfunction; that is, the image of preventing future dysfunction is not in the minds of most people attracted to the mental health field.

Many professionals whose livelihood and status are largely dependent on treatment do not welcome the idea of prevention. They are the first to cry that prevention is pie in the sky and simply diverts needed funds away from programs for the sick and disabled. They insist that primary prevention is fantasy, despite evidence to the contrary. As I mentioned at the beginning of the chapter, prevention efforts are far from fantasy in a growing number of states, including Michigan, Ohio, California, North Carolina, and Georgia.

In Michigan, for example, the Division of Prevention and Indirect Services of the state mental health department has established programs in hospitals and clinics to promote bonding between mothers and infants—which, as we have seen, is an important step in preventing later disturbed parent-child relationships and child abuse. The prevention division also offers services to children whose parents are in mental hospitals or receiving psychiatric treatment. Social support networks, such as those we mentioned earlier, are used to help these children. A third program is being developed for children whose parents are divorcing. For adults, courses in parenting are being instituted at community mental health centers, along with stress management training.

In Ohio, the section on primary prevention in the Department of Mental Health is also offering services through community mental health centers and other agencies to children whose parents are in the process of divorce.

In California, a primary prevention program in Madera County has focused on raising self-esteem, along with grade point average and attendance, of high school students in five schools. Courses in values clarification and communication skills were offered an experimental group of students in five schools. Compared with students in a control group, significant differences were found at the end of the program in both self-esteem and attendance.

The recently formed office of prevention in the California mental health division is setting up guidelines for prevention programs to be offered by community mental health centers and is emphasizing the need for evaluation. Chuck Roppel, director of the office, is convinced that prevention strategies can be designed so that "you can prove that prevention works." He does not believe, as I do not, that major mental illness, in the form of schizophrenia or manic-depressive psychosis, can be prevented at this time, since these are probably genetically related. He notes, however, that the great majority of cases seen at community mental health centers are problems of living that are causing people much pain and distress, and many of these can be prevented.

In North Carolina, a number of plans and activities are under way to start making primary prevention a reality in that state. Actually, as Ruth Relos, director of the office of prevention, points out: "There have been prevention programs operating for some time, but they haven't been called that." One program identifies mothers at high risk for potential child abuse and makes appropriate interventions. Another deals with preventing overreactions to floods and other natural disasters. Relos is also convinced that much mental distress can be prevented—distress connected with such problems as divorce, hypertension, or having a child with a terminal illness. Again, careful evaluation will be necessary so that results can be demonstrated.

ATTACKING MULTIPLE FACTORS

In Georgia, a prevention unit within the Division of Mental Health and Mental Retardation has been in operation for some four years. A Life Skills for Mental Health program has been going on for three years and has reached some 100,000 students throughout the state. It teaches stress management, decision making, relating to others, and valuing self. Instruments to evaluate outcome are now being tested. Some of the outcome measures will be changes in the number of behavioral problems, attendance record, and self-esteem. Other activities sponsored by the prevention unit include an anticipatory guidance program that offers classes on divorce and coupling and is based on a stress model. In one city, an alcoholism prevention program is underway.

Maury Weil, director of the unit, said that since a genetic relationship has been fairly well established for schizophrenia, a series of family planning programs will be offered in an attempt to reduce the incidence of this problem. He notes that effective prevention of mental health problems depends on narrowing one's focus so that "global" approaches are not being used. Most mental health problems involve a number of factors—social, psychological, environmental, biological—and the key to an effective strategy is separating these out and attacking one at a time. And the key to effective evaluation depends on a similar narrowing of focus.

Sixteen years ago, President Kennedy (1963) called for a bold new approach to mental health based on prevention. Until fairly recently, his message was largely ignored, and primary prevention continued to be rhetoric rather than reality. Despite the obstacles of few funds and recalcitrant attitudes, we now have solid evidence that prevention is both possible and feasible, provided nonglobal approaches are used and stringent criteria are followed. In view of the programs that have already demonstrated results, and the growing efforts in several states, we may well be on the threshold of making primary prevention a fact that will touch the lives of an increasing number of people.

References

BLOOM, B. L. A university freshman preventive intervention program: Report of a pilot project. *Journal of Consulting and Clinical Psychology*, 1971, *37*, 235-242.

BROUSSARD, E. R. Primary prevention program for new born infants at high risk for emotional disorder. In D. C. Klein and S. E. Goldston (Eds.), *Primary prevention: An idea whose time has come.* Washington, DC: Government Printing Office, 1977.

COBB, S. Social support as a moderator of life stress. *Psychosomatic Medicine,* 1976, *38,* 300-314.

GOLDSTON, S. E. An overview of primary prevention programming. In D. C. Klein and S. E. Goldston (Eds.), *Primary prevention: An idea whose time has come.* Washington, DC: Government Printing Office, 1977.

HEBER, R., & GARBER, H. The Milwaukee Project: A study of the use of family intervention to prevent cultural-familial mental retardation. In B. Z. Friedlander et al. (Eds.), *The exceptional infant: Assessment and intervention.* New York: Brunner/Mazel, 1975.

HOLLISTER, W. G. Basic strategies in designing primary prevention programs. In D. C. Klein and S. E. Goldston (Eds.), *Primary prevention: An idea whose time has come.* Washington, DC: Government Printing Office, 1977.

KENNEDY, J. F. *Message from the President of the United States relative to mental illness and mental retardation* (88th Congress, First Session). Washington, DC: Government Printing Office, 1963.

KENNEL, J., VOSS, D., & KLAUS, M. Parent-infant bonding. In R. Helfer and C. H. Kempe (Eds.), *Child abuse and neglect: The family and the community.* Cambridge, MA: Ballinger, 1976.

KLEIN, D. C., & GOLDSTON, S. E. (Eds.) *Primary prevention: An idea whose time has come.* Washington, DC: Government Printing Office, 1977.

LAMB, H. R., & ZUSMAN, J. Primary prevention in perspective. *American Journal of Psychiatry,* 1979, *136,* 12-17.

MUNOZ, R. F. The primary prevention of psychological problems. *Community Mental Health Review,* 1976, *1,* 1-15.

MUNOZ, R. F., & KELLY, J. G. *The prevention of mental disorders.* Homewood, IL: Richard D. Irwin, 1975.

The President's Commission on Mental Health. Report of the task panel on prevention, Volume IV. Washington, DC: Government Printing Office, 1978.

SILVERMAN, P. R. Widowhood and preventive intervention. *The Family Coordinator,* 1972, *21,* 95-102.

SKIPPER, J. K., & LEONARD, R. C. Children, stress, and hospitalization: A field experiment. *Journal of Health and Social Behavior,* 1968, *9,* 275-287.

SPIVACK, G., & SHURE, M. Preventively oriented cognitive education of preschoolers. In D. C. Klein and S. E. Goldston (Eds.), *Primary prevention: An idea whose time has come.* Washington, DC: Government Printing Office.

Part V

ISSUES IN SERVICE DELIVERY

Chapter 11

EVOLVING STRATEGIES

WILLIAM G. HOLLISTER

In the last 25 years, we have literally shared in the creation and implementation of an entirely new, supplementary system of mental health care in this country. Building upon the legacies of the 100 years of the "Dorothea Dix era" of state hospital programs, we as a nation have now added many kinds of new and complementary community systems of care, all as a nationwide effort to make more care available to those who need it. Through our collective efforts, the "community era" of care has arrived, not only for the mentally ill but also for the mentally retarded, alcoholics, and substance abusers as well.

Although the past 25 years have been a time of enormous growth for public mental health, this change was facilitated by a number of earlier developments, e.g., the establishment of child guidance clinics and psychopathic hospitals in the early part of the century, the casualty management experiences of World War II, advances in psychiatric epidemiology, and the establishment of the National Institute of Mental Health. These antecedent developments will be covered in other chapters. This chapter will consider selected key changes that have occurred in several operational areas of mental health programming: service delivery strategy, treatment modalities, consultation strategies, prevention methods, education interventions, and administrative processes.

CHANGES IN SERVICE DELIVERY STRATEGY AND SCOPE

During these years our service delivery strategy has moved far beyond caring for the relatively few persons sent to state hospitals, the ill who could not be socially tolerated. We have begun a growing commitment, not yet attained or fully accepted, of trying to provide services for individuals with all kinds of disorders at all levels of severity. This more comprehensive commitment to all who may be ill (Brown & Cain, 1964), including not only severe illness but also milder disorders, as has always been done in physical medicine, has been motivated both by professional and community compassion and by an increasing documentation that mental health competencies are relevant and needed to serve these people. Unfortunately, this broader definition as to whom we are to serve has provoked within our profession as internal tension between those who visualize the responsibilities of our field as covering a wide range of psychosocial and biological problems versus those who fear the dilution of overcommitment and recommend a focus only on the mentally ill (Langsley, 1980). A progressive increase in public expectations, demands, and in legislative fiats, plus our own desires to merit public trust and financial support, have led us through a series of expansions of our mandate and programs (Joint Commission on Mental Illness and Health, 1961). This conceptual change, this responsibility to provide a broader range of services, has induced a host of secondary changes, propelling us into some of the profound changes in consultation, prevention, education, and administration that will be discussed below.

CHANGES IN TREATMENT MODALITIES

The early 1950s saw an increase in interest in psychological processes as key factors in human behavioral disabilities, although some persisted in focusing on biological causes and solutions. The advent of psychopharmacological tools has dramatically swung the pendulum back toward more of a balance in the use of biological and psychological treatment methods. However, even as our treatment capabilities and resources to handle acute illness increased and our ability to return some of the chronically ill back to community life improved, we became more sensitive to the secondary social deterioration that accompanies the emotional isolation and alienation of the mentally ill (Goffman, 1961; Gruenberg et al., 1966). We came face to face with the fact that our psychotherapeutic and biological interventions were not enough to cope with the social disability in some of our patients. Bitterly stung by the catastrophe of premature deinstitutionalizations, perhaps one of the greatest errors of the past 25 years, we are now working hard to strengthen and expand our comparatively neglected social and emotional rehabilitation resources, shifting over from "pill centered" aftercare to community support programs for the chronically disabled.

Just as this has been happening to alter our armamentarium of interventions, another change has been occurring: the public's utilization of our Community Mental Health Center treatment programs. Although our collective group of community mental health centers are treating more psychotics and neurotics than ever before, there has been a profound shift in the kind of problems the public brings to us for care. As Bass and Ozarin (1977) have pointed out, the centers' case loads are now predominantly made up of individuals presenting situational disorders, behavior disorders, relationship breakdowns, and/or stress reactions–problems involving more moderate or mild levels of disability.

Faced with declining financial support, the inability to recruit clinicians, and a rising volume of admissions, more and more centers have begun exploring the use of nonclinical treatment modalities. In a search for the most parsimonious yet effective care (Hollister & Rae-Grant, 1972), they are selecting patients for "time trials" with clinical problem-oriented kinds of mental health education, or time trials at group experiences, or membership in emotional support or self-help groups. An increased use of activity and sheltered work experiences is emerging in the form of group living or home care programs and other less-than-direct clinical care approaches. Mental retardation programs and substance abuse programs, in their move to avoid institutionalization and to manage their patients in the community, are turning to the use of advocates and case managers to provide long-term or even lifetime medical, housing, activity, life support, and personal services to the chronically disabled.

All this shift in the types of services and treatments offered has brought about significant changes in the make-up of the service staffs. Today's center staff includes not only the clinically trained mental health professionals but also a large number of counselors, aides, educators, group home staff, case managers, group process specialists, and other personnel. Profound changes in mandate, utilization, treatment resources available, and the balance of disciplines on the staff are occurring in our mental health centers. As the range of patients and clientele expands, so has the range of interventions used (Miller et al., 1978).

CHANGES IN CONSULTATION AS A STRATEGY OF SERVICE DELIVERY

As epidemiological studies have demonstrated, a significant proportion of the unserved population with mental health needs do not or will not seek the help they need from mental health agencies (Regier et al., 1978). Thus, consultation has risen in importance as a service delivery strategy. It has become apparent that our former passive, receptive stance of waiting for people to define themselves as patients and be willing to come to us fails to access many of those in need or to provide comprehensive services to our catchment areas. As a result, we have moved out into the community to reach people where they are taking their problems. We find that other human service agencies are carrying large case loads of multiproblem cases, some of whose problems are recognizably mental health-related.

In these years, we have moved beyond merely providing case-centered consultations toward providing a more extensive range of consultee consultation services. This change is part of a strategy to build up and strengthen a "front line of agencies, professionals, and programs" so they will be capable of more competently managing many of the mild- and moderate-level mental health problems that are an expectable part of their daily service loads. Thus, informal, on-call case consultations now frequently evolve into regular consultee-centered and/or program development consultations that may be supplemented by training, diagnostic evaluation, and progress appraisal services. These are often formalized into ongoing interagency relationships by contracts. Consultation has matured into being a key skill of mental health professionals and a key component of comprehensive mental health community services (Caplan, 1970).

CHANGES IN PREVENTION

Changes in the development and methods of prevention have been late in arriving. Despite the early victories in eliminating the monoetiological disorders such as paresis, pellagra, and various toxic psychoses, the prevention of the various psychological disorders fell into a doldrums in its development. Its realization has been slowed by professional scoffing, the acute need to focus resources on the very ill, and by premature demands that prevention prove itself before it has had a chance to mature its technologies to prevent multietiological disorders. In contrast, it is interesting to note that we gave psychotherapy 40 years to mature before insisting it be evaluated. As result, prevention has received only desultory support at the governmental and professional level.

Recently, a real change appears to be occurring, especially at the grass roots level, where many small, low-cost prevention activities are being explored, based more on practical common sense than on preestablished scientific proof. With the advent of the "stress paradigm" as a conceptual model, many have found program design a much easier operation. By devising ingenious ways to lower the stressor loads on people at risk, to help persons avoid exposure to stressors, or to build up coping mechanisms or emotional resilience in times of crisis, innovative services are being tested and evaluated (Hollister, 1977). Prevention technology is maturing by first learning how to meet limited goals, leaving the prevention of the major disabilities until later, just as prevention in physical medicine has done.

New modes of preventive interventions are being forged and evaluated, for example, interventions that prevent role failures, relationship breakdowns, and psychobiological stress reactions (Cowen, 1977). Interventions are being designed to protect vulnerable persons, anticipate and prepare for expectable life crises, and to promote psychological growth and the capacity to cope with or endure stress. Prevention is undergoing a change whose time has come. For different perspectives, see the chapters by Lemkau and Justice elsewhere in this volume.

CHANGES IN EDUCATIONAL INTERVENTIONS

Mental health education has also risen from the ashes of disuse and rejection during the past 25 years. Not too long ago, educational interventions were considered ineffectual and evanescent, as mere "conceptual engrams" incapable of impacting the deep unconscious processes that govern people's behavior. Today, thanks to research on the learning process and operant conditioning, and thanks to research and experience with group therapy and group process, we now accept more fully that learning can be emotional as well as cognitive, that emotional reeducation is possible, and that behaviors can be unlearned or relearned. Today, many blends of group therapy and group educational experiences and services abound. Some mental health centers are selectively placing certain of their clientele into "time trials" at individual or group education on clinical problem-oriented topics in order to develop understandings and explore new behavior choices, either as a supplement or an alternative to psychotherapy. During these 25 years, professional rejection has turned to more serious study of education's role in behavior change (National Committee for Mental Health Education, 1977).

ADMINISTRATIVE CHANGES

Finally, there have been those needed, but sometimes painful, developments we have had to make in the administrative sphere. By critical and trenchant demands emanating from legal, social, and political sources, we have literally wrenched out of our former casual and second priority viewpoints about administration. Through sharp critiques, financial threats, and legal fiats we have been confronted with the need to put our houses in order and to adopt more up-to-date concepts of management (Feldman, 1973).

Today, we march to quite different administrative drummers. Heightened by the necessity to achieve more responsible use of public funds and to protect human rights, the entire health industry now must carefully assess needs, establish priorities, and develop its plans in concert with community voices (PL94-63). Our deliberations and operations must now be more open to community review and participation. We must more fully accept public accountability for the funds we use and the staff resources we expend. Management by objectives, management information and record systems, regular employee work and clinical supervision, employee appraisal and employee development programs, periodic program review and outcome evaluations, as well as quality of care assessments and human rights reviews, are now a part of our service-giving. These momentous demands, which take so much time and effort in the face of declining budgets and increasing service loads, have produced much stress in us. This is a change still in progress that will demand further balancing and development.

There is currently strong concern over the reality that we have not yet been able to access and serve some of the most vulnerable and needy segments of our population. We have also encountered much difficulty achieving the kinds of interagency and interdisciplinary collaboration deemed desirable. Some are proposing that mental health be subsumed under general medicine and/or broad human services agencies. Some administrative realignments are being field tested and evaluated.

SUMMARY

Finally, any review of the changes in our field has to consider the change in the mental health personnel involved. Have we changed? One might say we have become "sadder but wiser." I sense that we have grown considerably. Thanks to better training programs and stronger supplementary in-service training, I think we are better prepared, more capable, and more flexible service providers. We have become more community-oriented, more organizationally minded. The 1960s helped many of us become more sensitive to human rights, to the needs of women, various races, and minorities.

To have survived and succeeded in these halcyon years, we had to become more pluralistic, more humanistic, and more open to the contributions of many disciplines and professions. We have had to accept more fully that at its core, mental health is essentially an interdisciplinary agency and multiple intervention field of endeavor requiring the sensitive collaboration of many disciplines, agencies, and approaches.

Personally, I hope that all these momentous changes have not extinguished our desire to keep mental health services personalized and humanized, that we have not fallen into the trap of being mechanical and manipulative. Most of all, I hope we have learned better how to get along with one another, and how to model the kind of mentally healthy relationships that we try to provide for those we serve.

The principal lesson from this retrospective look at these evolving strategies is the realization that the change process set in motion has only begun. It still remains incomplete in many dimensions. We have not yet attained the goals of "comprehensiveness of services," nor have we provided easy access for all in need. We are still struggling to determine, by research and clinical evaluations, what the most appropriate care is for each kind of person and each kind of problem for which people request our assistance. Our concept of what the best utilization of our manpower is merits further study. There is still a conceptual lag between how preservice education resources are preparing our future manpower and the kind of knowledge skills and performance demands they need to carry out community services. In the face of budget cuts and rising case loads, the resources to do program evaluations, quality-of-care monitoring, and continuous need assessments; to develop consultation, education, and prevention programs; and to organize nonclinical community support services are being sharply reduced or eliminated, despite their essential value.

Most of all, we have not yet solved the problem of how to make our services effectively and truly "community" governed, financed, and utilized. It is hard for us to move beyond the professional benevolence of putting "psychiatry into the community" to the evocative task of achieving a real psychiatry of and by the community. We still struggle between whether we should provide "community services for the mentally ill" or "community mental health services," or both. We still depend too much on professional appeals and concern for the sick as the leverages with which to win financial support, yet devote little time and effort to the long-range task of building a community constituency to help guarantee our financial futures.

In sum, the change process is in vital need of continuation, repair, and extension, as well as renewed dedication to its original goals. It needs to be fortified with new objectives and methodologies to ensure its progress. The strategies for the delivery of community mental health services are still evolving.

References

BASS, R. D., & OZARIN, L. D. Community mental health center program: What is past is prologue. Paper presented at the annual meeting of the American Psychiatry Association, Toronto, Canada, May 1977.

BROWN, B. S., & CAIN, H. Many meanings of "comprehensive": Key issues in implementing President Kennedy's Program. *American Journal of Orthopsychiatry*, 1964, *34*, 834-839.

CAPLAN, G. *The theory and practice of mental health consultation.* New York: Basic Books.

COWEN, E. L. Baby steps toward primary prevention. *American Journal of Community Psychiatry*, 1977, *5*,(1), 1-19.

FELDMAN, S. (Ed.) *The administration of mental health service.* Springfield, IL: Charles C. Thomas, 1973.

GOFFMAN, E. *Asylums.* Garden City, NY: Doubleday, 1961.

GRUENBERG, E. M., BRANDEN, S., & KASINS, R. V. Identifying cases of the social breakdown syndrome. *Milbank Memorial Fund Quarterly*, 1966, *41*, 150-155.

HOLLISTER, W. G. Basic strategies in designing primary prevention programs. In D. C. Klein and S. E. Goldston (Eds.), *Primary prevention: An idea whose time has come.* Washington, DC: Government Printing Office, 1977.

HOLLISTER, W. G., & RAE-GRANT, Q. The principles of parsimony in mental health center operations. *Canada's Mental Health*, 1972, *20*, 18-24.

Joint Commission on Mental Illness and Health. *Action for mental health.* New York: Basic Books, 1961.

LANGSLEY, D. G. The community mental health center: Does it treat patients? *Hospital & Community Psychiatry,* 1980, *31,* 815-819.

MILLER, F. T., MAZADE, N. A., MULLER, S., & ANDRULIS, D. Trends in mental health programming. *American Journal of Community Psychology,* 1978, *61,* 191-198.

National Committee for Mental Health Education. Personal communication, 1977.

REGIER, D. A., GOLDBERG., I. D., & TAUBE, C. A. The de facto U.S. mental health services system. *Archives of General Psychiatry,* 1978, *35,* 685-693.

Chapter 12

HEALTH/MENTAL HEALTH INTEGRATION

JULES V. COLEMAN

The goal of integrating mental health services in general health care has always been difficult and elusive; it has not become less so with the rapidly increased growth of the medical specialties, including psychiatry, since the early 1950s. This is hardly surprising in view of the distancing practices traditionally observed between psychiatry and the rest of medicine. However, as both have come to recognize the biopsychosocial unity of man in health and disease, they have become increasingly interested in bridging the biological and psychosocial for the sake of better patient care and have looked for workable linkages between the two areas of practice (Engel, 1980).

Efforts to bring psychiatric practice into the mainstream of medical care have included the introduction of psychiatric liaison services into general hospitals and the increasing use of psychiatric consultation by other physicians, the psychiatric education of medical students and practicing physicians, and more recently the integration of mental health services into institutional primary care programs. This many-fronted psychiatric outreach to hospital and ambulatory medical care has taken place for the most part in the last three decades and was made possible by the rapid growth in the number of psychiatrists and of departments of psychiatry in hospitals and medical schools.

The importance of integrating health/mental health services is highlighted by studies of the number and percentage distribution of persons with mental disorders by type of treatment setting in this country in 1975 (Regier et al., 1978). It was reported here that 60 percent of all persons with a mental disorder were seen in the so-called "primary care/outpatient medical sector," including office-based physicians, neighborhood health centers, and general hospital outpatient clinics and emergency rooms. In another study (USDHEW, 1978), it was reported that as of January 1976, non-Federal general hospitals maintained 791 inpatient psychiatric units, 703 outpatient psychiatric services, and 176 day treatment programs for psychiatric patients. Veterans Administration general hospitals added another 89 inpatient psychiatric units, 91 outpatient, and 59 day treatment psychiatric programs. These general hospital psychiatric services accounted for 20 percent of the inpatient episodes in all speciality mental health facilities in 1975.

However, the overall role of general hospitals in providing mental health services is much larger than that of their specialty psychiatric services. For example, discharges from non-Federal general hospital psychiatric units numbered 516,000 in 1975, whereas discharges with a primary psychiatric diagnosis from all general hospitals numbered 1,494,000, almost an additional 1 million discharges with a primary psychiatric diagnosis from general hospitals over and above those discharges from their specialty psychiatric units. If one adds discharges from general hospitals with a secondary diagnosis of mental disorder, it makes a total of 2.5 million of the 34 million discharges from non-Federal general hospitals, or 7 percent of the total with a primary or secondary diagnosis of mental disorder.

There was an increase of 42 percent in discharges with a primary diagnosis of mental disorder between 1971 and 1975, compared with an increase of 16 percent in total discharges from general hospitals. The number of discharges with a secondary but not a primary diagnosis of mental disorder increased 52 percent during the same period. The prominence of psychiatric diagnoses in the general hospital picture presumably reflects an increase in the number of psychiatric units in general hospitals over the years. The differential increase in secondary psychiatric diagnoses may be related to the increasing liaison role of psychiatric departments with medical-surgical departments, as well as a continued increase in insurance coverage for mental disorders.

Liaison Psychiatry. Lipowski (1979) describes liaison psychiatry in a medical setting as the "regular contact by a psychiatrist or other mental health worker with the clinical staff for the purpose of enhancing psychosocial aspects of patient care." He goes on to say: "Such liaison involves participation in ward rounds and meetings, and mediation between patients and staff to prevent disruptions of care by interpersonal conflicts and inadequate communication. Furthermore, efforts are made to sensitize staff members to those psychological and social issues that add to the burden of illness and to the stress of taking care of them for the staff." From the point of view of relations among different medical specialties, this is a somewhat prickly concept, since it implies that psychiatrists and their co-workers play superordinate educational and mediating roles with respect to the professional activities of other specialties.

Liaison psychiatry proposes to introduce collaborative methods in dealing with the psychosocial as well as the physical problems of medical care. However, true collaboration as a partnership of equals encounters serious difficulties because of the hierarchic status concepts of most physicians in the medical and surgical specialties, as well as in psychiatry. Undergraduate and graduate medical education indoctrinates students with the importance of a sense of personal responsibility and of unquestioning self-confidence. Physicians are trained to regard the doctor-patient relationship as a private contract in which their obligation is only toward individual patients. The hierarchic social role is strengthened in medical students and house officers by the use of teaching hospitals for clinical training and experience where professional models strongly support such a role (Dingwell, 1980).

Efforts to implement a genuinely collaborative, biopsychosocial approach to patients run into many obstacles, including the resistance of physicians (Greenhill, 1977), differences between physically and psychologically minded physicians (Watson, 1966), and the resistance of doctors to the disorganizing and distressing effects of information overload in confronting the complex and unfamiliar demands of understanding psychosocial factors in illness (Lipowski, 1974). The latter underscores the differences between the clinical orientation of medical practice and the psychosocial orientation required to understand a patient's personal and social experiences as they relate to his or her illness. Clinicians work to isolate the situations they encounter with the aim of controlling the conditions of treatment. Treatment by physicians is based on an authoritative view of their role in which they expect their "orders" to be followed explicitly. In contrast, a holistic frame of reference, congenial to collaborative practice, regards the patient as an integrated component of a family and social context, participating in making decisions based on an understanding of his or her reactions to the threats of illness and medical treatment (Coleman, 1981).

The goal of comprehensive medical care on the basis of a collaborative biopsychosocial model might seem more easily realized in the community, outside the hospital and the traditionally rigid hierarchy of inpatient medical treatment. We shall now examine a number of community programs and a variety of health/mental health interactions.

Consultation. A patient is referred to a mental health worker by another health professional for diagnosis, evaluation, feedback, and discussion or written report with recommendations. Too often, the referring physician gets no feedback or uniformative notes of acknowledgment. The long-range value of consultation for the referring person, from the point of view of health/mental health integration, depends on a continuing professional relationship between the referring source and the mental health consultant, the availability of the consultant for informal and emergency consultation, and mutual agreement on the consultative objectives.

The North Carolina Project. This program met these conditions. It was a consultation program with a specific objective, namely, to assist community physicians in the aftercare of patients discharged from a public mental hospital (Stratas & Cathell, 1966). The project was developed in 1961 under the auspices of the North Carolina Department of Mental Health with the aim of bringing psychiatric care to some of the 4 million persons who lived at the time in rural and semirural areas without psychiatric resources. It was intended to help community physicians in their work with ex-hospital patients.

The plan was to use the regional mental hospital as a home base from which a psychiatrist would travel two and a half days a week to certain rural counties to visit local physicians. It was expected that as the psychiatrist developed working relations with the physicians through consultations on aftercare patients, he would be in a position to advise them about other emotionally disturbed patients and about general psychosocial problems they encountered in their practice.

The psychiatrist did a good deal of preparation, studying, and visiting the five project counties, exploring their unique community patterns, their power structures, the interactions among their agencies, and the relationship of the local physicians to these agencies. The psychiatrist established separate consultative relations with each of the local 58 physicians in the project, visiting them in their offices and making it clear that he was there to help, not to take patients over. He set up mutually convenient times to meet with each of the physicians and followed their lead in making consultative arrangements. He established a regular route, a copy of which was sent to each physician each month. He encouraged them to contact him by telephone at any time, and this ready availability did much to persuade the doctors to accept responsibility for treating patients they would formerly automatically refer to special treatment centers.

The project was considered a success. It demonstrated that with psychiatric support, community physicians could take care of even the most disturbed patients living in a community. One of the counties in the project soon significantly decreased the number of patients it sent to the state hospital. Psychiatric admissions to local general hospitals increased from 10 percent of all admissions to 30 percent during the project, with patients assigned to general medical wards.

The project was finally terminated, apparently having served its demonstration purpose. Such a project could probably be established and maintained at the present time through third-party payments for the work of the psychiatrist. An important consideration for its continuing support would be an administrative structure covering a number of such undertakings, supplying training resources, manpower, recruitment, a clearing house function for the exchange of information, and substitute coverage as needed.

The Minnesota Project. Undertaken at about the same time, this project was established in a rural area of Minnesota by Kiesler (1975), who accepted the position with the stipulation that he would not take on any patients for treatment but would devote his time entirely to consultation and indirect service, assisting physicians in the area to carry out the mental health care of their patients. Since there were no other psychiatrists in the area, he was able to carry on his program with satisfactory results for more than twelve years. Over time, there developed increasing pressure by the physicians for the consultant to treat patients, and this has been done in recent years.

Both the North Carolina and the Minnesota Programs required that the psychiatrist as consultant take into account the special problems of community physicians and their capacity for long-term care of psychiatrically disturbed patients. Both programs presupposed the continuing, reliable involvement of the psychiatrist with the same physicians over an indefinite period of time. Psychiatric consultation with physicians, but without the opportunity to have their patients seen and possibly treated by mental health personnel, does seem to have limitations for many physicians and possibly to lead to dissatisfaction.

Cooperative arrangements between health and mental health programs presuppose that the mental health program is an established administrative component of an overall health service. The President's Commission on Mental Health, in its report submitted to the White House in April 1978, proposed that such working arrangements should allow for:

(1) mental health personnel to provide direct care and treatment in the health care setting to patients with emotional disorders whose problems exceed the skills of nonpsychiatric health care providers;

(2) consultation directed toward altering behavior patterns that increase the risk of physical illness;
(3) collaborative treatment with nonpsychiatric health care practitioners for those patients with combined physical and mental illness; and
(4) training nonpsychiatric physicians and other health care personnel to enhance their skills in the treatment of patients with relatively mild emotional disorders.

These recommendations are of interest; however, they underrate the ability of primary care personnel to take care of a wide range of psychiatric problems, from the very mild to the very severe (Coleman & Patrick, 1978).

Because of the pluralistic nature of health care in this country, it is generally agreed that implementing the coordination of the mental health and general health care systems will require a number of conceptual organizational models. The three principal types of health care delivery in this country are fee-for-service, prepaid practice, and community or neighborhood health centers. In fee-for-service health care, the importance of the mental health component has been most readily recognized and accepted in pediatrics. It is estimated that 80 percent of pediatricians make at least some effort to practice a behavioral approach in the belief that it is an integral part of reasonable, even minimal, primary care and must be recognized as such (Pakula, 1979).

In prepaid health care, as exemplified by health maintenance organizations (HMOs), subscribers enter into a contractual arrangement with the provider agency to pay a prearranged amount for the agreed upon medical services. Federally funded HMOs are required to provide enrollees with up to 20 visits a year to mental health clinicians, along with unlimited visits to primary physicians for treatment of emotional problems. Most HMOs have set up separate psychiatric clinics for subscribers within their organization or have purchased specialized psychiatric services outside the plan, following the traditional separation of health and mental health services in this country. Community or neighborhood health centers are structured much like prepaid health plans, except that comprehensive medical care is provided to a geographically defined population. Almost all employ salaried physicians. These centers are largely subsidized by public funds and provide free or low-cost services to economically disadvantaged and medically underserved persons.

Primary health care is defined as "accessible, comprehensive, coordinated, and continual care by accountable providers of health services" (National Academy of Sciences, 1978). Primary care providers include general practitioners, family practitioners, internists, pediatricians, and often specialists in obstetrics/gynecology for patients in the childbearing years. It has been estimated that 60 percent of all persons with mental disorder in this country were seen in the "primary care/outpatient sector" (Regier et al., 1978). Of patients seen by primary care providers, a series of reports in various countries indicates that about 15-25 percent present evidence of mental disorder (Shepherd et al., 1966; Hoeper, 1979; Patrick et al., 1978). There is also considerable evidence that primary care physicians on their own identify only about 2 percent of their emotionally disturbed patients (Hoeper, 1979). When mental health and primary care services are integrated professionally, administratively, and structurally, there is improved case identification, particularly when mental health workers are located physically in the primary care work areas (Coleman & Patrick, 1976). Devices for screening mental disorders may also improve case identification (Goldberg et al., 1969).

Medical utilization, that is, the number of care-seeking visits per patient per year, is greatly influenced by the presence of emotional disorders, and patients with chronic or nonchronic emotional disturbances use medical services much more frequently than do patients without emotional disorders (Patrick et al., 1978; Tessler et al., 1976).

Identification of mental disorders in a primary care setting might seem to serve little purpose without the availability of treatment resources. However, there is some evidence that when primary care clinicians are made aware of emotional problems in patients, the problems seem to respond more quickly. In a study reported by Johnstone and Goldberg (1976), results of psychiatric screening showing clear evidence of problems in patients rated as normal by their doctors were discussed with the doctors; a control group was set up where the results were withheld from the doctors. Patients in the control group gradually improved with time, but with an average of 5.3 illness-months following initial consultation, in contrast to 2.8 illness-months for the patients whose disorder had been discussed with their doctor. Studies of this kind are informative. One still asks: To what extent can primary care physicians treat patients with emotional problems? What kinds of problems need to be referred for specialized mental health treatment? There are many questions and currently few answers. If primary care personnel underidentify, it may be that mental health personnel over-identify psychiatric problems, particularly the need for psychiatric treatment.

PRIMARY HEALTH CARE PROGRAMS

We shall discuss two major forms of primary care that provide "accessible, comprehensive, coordinated and continual care," including mental health services: HMOs and neighborhood health centers (NHCs). We might also mention primary care centers in general hospitals, a relatively recent development, often established for the purpose of providing non-emergency care in medicine and pediatrics, thus freeing emergency rooms for the care of more critical situations and of developing family health programs for training residents in family practice. Because of staff rotations, they are often unable to assign patients to their own clinicians on a continuing basis. Psychiatrists in these centers serve as consultants and educators. They are not involved in direct patient care but help providers to identify and treat the psychiatric problems of patients, and to increase staff awareness of how psychosocial factors influence the course of illness (Slaby et al., 1978; Schniewind, 1977).

Health maintenance organizations are prepaid group practices (PGPs) such as the Kaiser-Permanente Plans, which provide care in their own clinics or health centers, or they may be medical foundations or independent practice associations, which arrange for prepaid patients to be seen by physicians in their own private offices. Medical care foundations rarely establish ongoing cooperative arrangements with mental health services, and for this reason will not be discussed further. Prepaid group practices may become qualified for federal funding under the HMO Act of 1973 if they provide certain expanded services, including specified mental health services. Mental health services were not included in the basic health benefits of early PGPs but have since become a common component of comprehensive care in response to pressures brought by subscribers and by the attractions of federal qualification, which requires all organizations employing more than 25 persons to offer the option of their own health insurance package or membership in a federally qualified HMO if one is located in the area (Group for the Advancement of Psychiatry, 1980).

On the whole, PGPs have met with a good deal of subscriber satisfaction because they provide comprehensive medical care and continuity over long periods of time for all members of a family and because almost all health services are provided in a single health center. However, studies have indicated that 7 percent of patients were frankly dissatisfied with their services, and between 25 and 50 percent had used the services of non-plan physicians at one time or another. The primary reasons seemed to be difficulties in breaking established care patterns, delays in forming new relationships within the plan, inconveniences in appointment systems, transportation problems, interpersonal difficulties, and dislike of a "clinic" atmosphere (Weinerman, 1966: 232).

We shall discuss the PGP from the point of view of its efforts to include mental health services in primary health care, but first it must be emphasized that primary care clinicians are the basic mental health resource in PGPs as in other settings. They take care of about 70 percent of psychiatric patients on their own, referring the rest for mental health care. Referral depends not so much on the nature of the psychiatric diagnosis as on the time required for care and on the complexity of the management problem. Most PGP patients with diagnoses of schizophrenia or endogenous depression can be treated by primary clinicians if the necessary medication schedule has been established psychiatrically, or if patients respond well to the primary clinician's medication efforts (Coleman & Patrick, 1976).

At Kaiser-Permanente in Santa Clara, California, an experimental systems approach to mental health care was carried out with the help of NIMH funding. The approach was based on early screening and identification of health problems through automated multiphasic health testing with a population of 5000 new members. After screening, all patients in the experimental group were informed in groups how to use the facilities of the plan and were then given a health education program. Four patient categories were identified (Garfield, 1970):

(1) well/well: no physical findings and no complaints;
(2) sick/well: significant findings but no complaints, as in hypertension;
(3) well/sick: no significant findings but some complaints—the "worried well";
(4) sick/sick: significant findings and complaints.

The well/sick were considered at risk for the development of mental health problems. They were examined by nurse clinicians who looked for evidence of psychological or emotional problems. If appropriate, patients were referred for treatment or education programs intended to help them deal more effectively with their perceptions about health and illness and to teach them to use social strategies other than physician visits or tranquilizers to reduce stress. The sick/sick were referred for appropriate traditional care. A special clinic was also set up for medical review of individuals with complex, interrelated physical, psychophysiological, and psychosocial problems. The program at Santa Clara is significant in that it introduces mental health services in an established HMO along the lines of the public health model of screening, case identification, establishment of a continuum of health services, and problem-oriented programs of health education.

It also has many of the drawbacks of the public health model with regard to psychiatric illnesses. Screening identifies psychopathology; it does not address itself to the patient's sense of himself or herself as ill, nor to his or her health-seeking motivation. These are matters for clinical evaluation and clinical judgement. For this reason, many primary physicians abjure screening and insist on doing their own initial evaluation of new patients, thus establishing the basis for an enduring doctor-patient relationship. However, the screening mentioned earlier, that is, through a brief health questions instrument (the General Health Questionnaire, reported on by Goldberg,1969), seems to have been found useful, and physicians might be interested in having their patients fill out the self-administered, brief questionnaire before the initial visit.

At the Community Health Care Center (CHCP) in New Haven, Connecticut, mental health services were integrated into primary care from the beginning, and there was no separate mental health clinic (Coleman & Patrick, 1976). The ideal of primary care/mental health collaboration was fostered by the development of small primary care teams. Each team consisted usually of two physicians, either internists or pediatricians, a physician assistant in adult medicine and a nurse practitioner in pediatrics, a mental health clinician, a medical assistant for each physician, and a receptionist. The mental health clinicians on the team were mostly psychiatric social workers, although one team had a clinical psychologist and another a psychiatric nurse practitioner. An important element in the plan was the willingness of primary care clinicians, with the support of mental health personnel, to accept responsibility for mental health problems as an essential component of comprehensive health services. Psychiatrists provided backup to primary care and mental health clinicians.

In actual practice, the teams achieved many of the objectives of a mini-psychiatric clinic, but unlike most psychiatric clinics, they treated all age groups and all complaints—physical, emotional, and social. Furthermore, cases were never closed and the medical record covered all conditions, at all times, as long as the patient was a member of the plan. The greater concentration of psychiatric expertise at a community psychiatric clinic is in general a myth, since the distribution of mental health personnel within a CHCC is not particularly different from that of most psychiatric clinics around the country. In favor of the health center is its emphasis on physical care, which we know is often a special problem among patients with psychiatric disorders. Also, all members of a family come to the center for their care, problems known to a family become known across team lines, and family planning or treatment is possible as the need arises (Coleman, 1981).

Neighborhood health centers are community-based facilities supported by public funding and devoted to the health care of poor or medically underserved populations. Originally funded by the Office of Economic Opportunity (OEO) and later by the Department of Health, Education and Welfare (DHEW), centers were established in communities in 42 states, serving an estimated 1.3 million people by 1974 (Walsh & Bicknell, 1977). Other sources of funding were developed by adding new services in such categorical programs as maternal and infant care, or children and youth projects.

These health centers have been sponsored by hospitals and medical schools more often than by local governments. Each has in common a family and community orientation with citizen participation at the board and staff paraprofessional levels, as well as an emphasis on continuity of care, service coordination, and team health care (Borus, 1976; Jacobson et al., 1978).

There have been many problems; the enthusiasms of the 1960s were followed by the budget retrenchments of the 1970s. There have also been conflicts over community control, difficulties in getting professionals to work in teams, high staff turnover, and in many instances, limits to the range of services provided. Nonetheless, the neighborhood health centers have done much to stimulate a new interest in primary care in this country, and most importantly, have helped to remove some of the barriers to health care for the poor and give the populations they serve an opportunity to participate in decisions about their health care (Group for the Advancement of Psychiatry, 1980).

The centers have approached the problem of providing mental health services in a number of ways, responding to the stimulation of citizen boards and the efforts of mental health professionals. Service models have ranged from that of hospital liaison/consultation psychiatry, to separate departments of mental health within a center, to interdisciplinary teams consisting of health, mental health, and social work personnel to coordinate planning and care and to facilitate interdepartmental referrals within the health center.

Neighborhood health centers have served as important experimental laboratories for testing health/mental health linkages, demonstrating the value of health/mental health programs for medically underserved populations, and for exploring health/mental health team approaches in providing comprehensive, coordinated, integrated health/mental health services to inner-city people. As laboratories, they have the advantage of providing opportunities for the exploration of alternative approaches, along with the disadvantage of depending on uncertain and potentially unreliable funding.

Health/Mental Health Linkages: A Summary of Conceptual Models. Pincus (1980) has outlined the major linkage models. Working arrangements or linkages between health and mental health services seek a variety of objectives, from that of facilitating the use of mental health services by interested patients to that of integrating health/mental health services so that they are inseparable components of an integrated health/mental health program. The following patterns or models are identified:

(1) Both systems, health and mental health, operate independently but with a formal or informal agreement between the two for patient referral, followup, or information transfer. The patient has the primary responsibility for making arrangements for psychiatric service. Examples are arrangements between a CMHC and private practitioners in the area (Borus, 1976) and CMHC-HMO linkages (USDHEW, 1974).

(2) *Triage:* Here again, an agreement is worked out between the two systems, but with two important differences: Generally, a more specific and articulated agreement is worked out, and a specifically designated staff person provides assessment and triage, thus easing the process of referral, information flow, and followup. This is a pattern developed between a community health center and a community mental health center (USDHEW, 1977).

(3) The general health center establishes its own mental health unit to provide evaluation and treatment of patients enrolled in the health program (Patterson, 1976; Goldensohn, 1972). This is the usual pattern of mental health services developed by most HMOs.

(4) An arrangement fashioned on the model of consultation/liaison services in general hospitals, where the emphasis is on mental health consultation, but with service provided by the consultants (Lipowski, 1974). The model is found in the pri-

mary care units of general hospitals (Lipowski, 1974; Rittlemeyer, 1978; Slaby et al., 1978). This approach emphasizes the educational values of consultation and often includes formal teaching provisions as well.

(5) *Supervision and Education.* Providing non-mental-health professionals with psychiatric knowledge and skills in dealing with the emotional problems of their own patients has been the emphasis of many programs (Rittlemeyer, 1972; Balint, 1957; Goldberg, 1979). Its success seems to be limited to the relatively small percentage of physicians who are attracted to such programs.

(6) *Integrated Health/Mental Health Teams.* In this model, a mental health professional becomes a continuing member of a health team, and there is no separate mental health department. All mental health activities go on between members of the team, including assessment, evaluation, consultation, referral, and education. The model has been described above for the Community Health Care Center in New Haven (Coleman & Patrick, 1976; Coleman 1977). It has also been developed in a Boston neighborhood health center (Morrill, 1977), and in a small family practice group in Canada (Adsett & Rudnick, 1978).

Health services in this country represent a pluralism of concept and practice. Changing times have witnessed new approaches to old problems and institutional adaptations to new economic, political, and cultural demands. Presumably, we have not come to the end of our restless search for new frontiers and new horizons. There are progressive forces that seek out change to serve new populations and new ideas, and there are conservative forces that resist change. The urge to introduce mental health into general health services is essentially a progressive force advocating individual right, need, and privilege. It is countered by forces that see the promise of human stability in the conservation of old values, and in the protective and stabilizing influences of institutional social processes such as education, religion, work, and the medical care system itself. With this in mind, but without further discussion of the problem of resistance to change, we shall now consider some of the special problems encountered in attempting to integrate health and mental health services.

Case Identification by Primary Physicians. As we have pointed out, it is estimated that 15-25 percent of patients in primary care practices show evidence of psychiatric problems. On the other hand, recognition of these problems varies enormously, from 2 to 39 percent, in individual practices (Hoeper, 1979; Goldberg, 1979), depending on the practitioner's level of interest and concern and his or her "psychiatric focus." It seems clear that few practitioners are interested in the psychosocial status of their patients. There is also little interest among practitioners in referrals to mental health clinicians (Sack, 1981). In two studies, one showed 0.9 percent and another 2.5 percent of all patients referred to psychiatrists; the first was a study of private practice internists (Shortell & Daniels, 1974), the second of physicians in a PGP (Locke et al., 1966).

Outcome Measures of Psychiatric Treatment in General Medical Practice. Treatment effectiveness is not easy to identify in psychiatry, except in conditions like manic states and endogenous depressions, where response to medication is often clear and sometimes dramatic. Certainly, the results of psychotherapy are not easy to assess, and outcome studies are by no means unambiguous in their findings (Bergin & Garfield, 1971). On the other hand, a number of studies have related mental health treatment, even of brief duration, to reductions in medical utilization (Cummings, 1977; Goldberg et al., 1970). Of interest also is a report (Cassem & Hackett, 1971) of 441 patients admitted to the coronary care unit at Massachusetts General Hospital during a 15-month period. The 145 patients seen in psychiatric consultation had a mortality rate of one-third that of the entire group. Reports of this kind are difficult to evaluate without more careful methodological considerations.

What happens to patients in primary practices who do not have the benefit of mental health considerations? What happens to patients who live in rural areas where there are no available mental health personnel? It should be noted that even in the best of circumstances, the availability of mental health providers will never saturate the potential treatment need, even if there were no physician or patient resistance and no fiscal barriers. There is, to be sure, evidence that over time many patients either get well spontaneously on their own or experience some moderation of their sufferings, or perhaps learn to adapt to their illness in such a way that it is no longer a particular burden (Ernst, 1959).

When all is said and done, referral for psychiatric treatment is by no means a guarantee that much benefit will ensue. In light of the high cost of the best possible psychiatric care, which will always be scarce, there is a great need to define more carefully what indications justify referral. This poses a dilemma, since there is a huge untapped reservoir of psychiatric cases among patients in the primary care system, where the likelihood of discriminating case-finding and referral is very small. From the point of view of psychiatry, the primary care sector represents a conglomeration of unsorted-out psychopathology that resists access and change.

If one differentiates chronic from nonchronic emotional problem patients, as we did in a study at CHCP (Patrick et al., 1978), one finds that the chronic represent 12.4 percent of patients with emotional problem complaints. It might be suggested: (1) that these patients should receive some psychiatric consideration, but (2) for the most part can be maintained by PCPs after psychiatric consultation. The problem is to unscramble the first group from the second, and this can probably only be done by a truly integrated, collaborative, health/mental health working arrangement (Coleman & Patrick, 1976).

Psychotherapy by the Primary Care Physician. A major source of information on the practice of psychotherapy by primary physicians comes from the experiences of the Canadian National Health Insurance program for psychiatric services (Richman & Brown, 1979: 177-205). The 1964 Report on the Royal Commission on Health Services recommended that: "Henceforth all discrimination and distinction between physical and mental illness in the organization and provision of service, the treatment, and the attitudes on which these discriminations are based, be disallowed for all times as unworthy and unscientific." The commission specified that the medical services benefit should incorporate insured medical services for the "diagnosis and treatment of all physical and psychiatric conditions including mental retardation." The "medicare" program did not change the delivery system, which continued to be provided by private practice physicians working on a fee-for-service basis. The patient has the choice of a physician, who submits a claim for an individual patient. The provincial data bases of individual hospitalization and medical services enable detailed studies of the use by the general population of specialized psychiatric services, mental health services from private practitioners, and general hospital care for mental disorders. In Saskatchewan, for example, 7 percent of psychiatric patients were seen by both psychiatrists and general practitioners; 77.8 percent were seen by general practitioners alone during 1971-72.

Not all general practitioners were equally interested in participating in the psychotherapy program. In Nova Scotia, among 500 general practitioners who earned more than $25,000 from the insurance program during 1977, 30 percent did not submit any claims for psychotherapy, and one-fourth submitted claims for less than $500 of psychotherapy during the year. The majority of psychotherapy in general practice was provided by a minority of practitioners. Of the 500 general practitioners, 38 physicians claimed 60 percent of the costs for general practitioner psychotherapy. Also of interest is that 2-4 percent of patients use 30-40 percent of mental health services.

What kinds of patients are treated by the primary physician? It has been pointed out that mental disorders must be differentiated from psychological and emotional reactions. Richman and Brown (1979) point out that it is difficult but necessary to differentiate among: (a) everyday personal reactions to everyday problems (temporary and appropriate reactions to stress); (b) problems of "emotionality," personality traits, and culturally determined behavior (subjective perceptions of "suffering"); (c) isolated psychological and behavioral symptoms and signs; and (d) syndromes for which there is good clinical consensus on their nature and severity, and considerable agreement on the type and amount of therapeutic intervention needed (Lewis, 1967).

Richman and Brown point out a second problem for clinical care, the *redistributive phenomenon.* In the development of prepaid health insurance programs, economists are concerned with the redistribution of medical resources from higher- to lower-income populations (Newhouse et al., 1974). It has been suggested that including psychiatry in health insurance programs may represent a subsidy to the rich from the poor (Albee, 1977; Crowell, 1977). However, it has also been suggested (McSweeney, 1977) that since psychotherapy is best suited to the needs of the well-educated and more affluent, provisions for psychotherapy in proposed national health insurance plans may benefit the relatively well-off at the expense of the general public.

Perhaps the most important consideration is that different services are needed by population groups with different economic and psychosocial needs, and that what many of the poor may require are psychotherapeutically oriented social services in addition to medical care. For example, in a study reported by Corney (1979), the extent of mental and physical ill health of clients referred to social workers in a local authority department and a general attachment scheme was examined. In both settings, a substantially high proportion were found to be suffering from ill health—physical, mental, or both. In other words, these were people who must evidently be classified in sociomedical or medicosocial terms if justice is to be done to their status (Shepherd, 1979).

In a study of chronic neurotic illness (Shepherd et al., 1979), it was possible to undertake a detailed analysis of a social worker's activities as related to clients' responses. In nearly two-thirds of the sample, the social worker's contribution was restricted to helping patients and their families to deal with practical problems and difficulties. In the remaining one-third, she exercised a quasi-psychotherapeutic function, although here too, practical help and support were often given (Baker, 1976). "The specificity of such intervention, however, remains questionable. On the available evidence the most probable explanation of any benefits conferred by the social worker appears to reside in the way in which her personal activities supplemented the resources which she mobilizes and which facilitate a more positive approach by the general practitioner towards a greater awareness of the social orbit of morbidity" (Shepherd, 1979).

Recognizing that when we speak of emotional problems, we mean psychological reactions to the social situation in which the patient is intimately involved, we might quote a prominent representative of the Royal College of Physicians (Crombie, 1972):

> The first thing a general practitioner has to decide is the relative importance of the emotional and physical factor in his patient's problems. Only the general practitioner approaches the matter quite in this way, and his ability to do so depends on his unique previous knowledge of the patient. Where this knowledge is denied to the doctor, assessment has to be made by more devious and less certain methods of evaluating the emotional component by exclusion of the organic. This method of evaluating the emotional component is clumsy. For the 10-20% of selected problems which reach the hospital-based doctor, it is unsuitable and also wasteful of medical resources. The organic element is less definable in illness encountered by general practitioners than it is in the selected illness encountered in hospital practice. The emotional element, on the other hand, is relatively more important in general practice.

The question of differences between the psychiatric populations of the primary care and the specialized psychiatric sectors has also been discussed by Shepherd (1979). He examines particularly the differences in depressed patients in the two populations and points out that the proportion of depressed patients who come to the attention of a psychiatrist is no more than 2.92 per 1000 of the general population and no more than 1.8 percent of all depressed people. This is in contrast to the estimated prevalence of depressed persons in the population, which according to Watts (1966) includes 12-15 persons per 1000 seen by general practitioners and perhaps as many as 150 persons per 1000 who do not consult any doctor. In this light, Shepherd (1979) states: "In consequence, psychiatrists in their clinical practice are familiar with only a very small band of the depressive spectrum, and one which differs in respect of presenting features and severity from the larger part."

CONCLUDING REMARKS

Cooperative arrangements between general health care and mental health personnel have been characterized by two major considerations. On the one hand, the goal has been to facilitate the referral of patients with psychiatric problems seen by general health practitioners to specialized psychiatric services. On the other, efforts have been made by mental health clinicians to find ways of working in general health care systems as consultants, educators, or collaborators, with the goal of introducing a mental health component into the general health care process in order to reach patients who would not ordinarily come within the purview of the psychiatric caretaking system.

In effect, we are dealing with two sets of mental health problems, one belonging to the general health and particularly the primary care system, the other to psychiatry, with a considerable area of overlap. Further, there is a mental health component in the primary care process which has as yet not received careful enough examination, although there seems little doubt that it differs radically from the mental health approach in psychiatry. It has been recognized that the primary care system is the major mental health resource in this country as elsewhere (Regier et al., 1978; Shepherd et al., 1966). One might thus reflect that there is little point in setting up a separate mental health network to take care of problems already receiving responsible attention from the primary care sector. In this connection Shepherd (1979), referring to the situation in Great Britain, has made the following remarks:

> Administrative and medical logic alike suggest that the cardinal requirement for improvement of the mental health services in this country is not a large expansion of psychiatric agencies, but rather a strengthening of the family doctor in his therapeutic role.

He recognizes that "family doctors have yet to play their potential role in the development of community mental health services" and suggests that their capacity to do so will depend on the next phase of the British health service, namely, the family doctor *team*, with the inclusion of nurses, health visitors, and eventually social workers. He further states:

> This approach is particularly suitable to the psychological aspects of ill health. It offers realistic prospects of achieving many of the objectives of the American community mental health centers with-

out the problems created by an extensive redistribution of manpower.

There are still many problems during this transition period in the growth of family practice as a major new specialty adding its strength to that of general internists and pediatricians in providing comprehensive medical care. We must keep in mind that only a small contingent of the primary care field (Richman & Brown, 1979) will be interested in doing psychotherapy in their practice. One must therefore be prepared to undertake intensive study of the mental health potentials of PCPs who are not interested in psychotherapy. What do they and what can they contribute to our area of interest?

If we follow Shepherd's reasoning, as applied to this country, we might regard the existing community mental health centers as a major potential resource for comprehensive health care by converting them stagewise into community or neighborhood health centers with a significant mental health component, and with the potential for the development of the family health teams referred to by Shepherd (1979). Integrated health/mental health teams, a group of professionals working together in the same physical location, serve the following mental health objectives (Coleman & Patrick, 1976): (1) case finding as a pathway to treatment; (2) treatment carried out mainly within the team; and (3) opportunities for informal discussion between health and mental health personnel of case management, referral, and feedback.

There are also two major general conflict areas which must be addressed: (1) working out ways to resolve problems created by conflicts arising from efforts to establish interprofessional collaboration; and (2) working out ways to resolve problems that arise between the small primary care team and overall administration.

The extension of the concept of comprehensive care to include integrated mental health services is the challenge of the next decade. It will require all our ingenuity, determination, and idealism to promote the objectives that we have learned from bitter experience are attended by interprofessional rivalries, problems of professional turf, and (in relation to our nonmedical professional colleagues) the issue of the dominant social and professional position of physicians. We have as yet no way of knowing how these issues can be resolved, but we do know that they must be resolved for a better health care system.

References

ADSETT, C. A., & RUDNICK, K. V. Psychiatric liaison with primary care team. *Psychiatric Opinion,* 1978, *15,* 29-33.

ALBEE, G. W. Does including psychotherapy in health insurance represent a subsidy to the rich from the poor? *American Psychologist,* 1977, *32,* 710-721.

BAKER, R. The multi-role practitioner in the generic orientation to social work practice. *British Journal of Social Work,* 1976, *6,* 327-352.

BALINT, M. D. *The doctor, his patient, and the illness.* New York: International Universities Press, 1957.

BERGIN, A. E., & GARFIELD, S. L. (Eds.) *Handbook of psychotherapy and behavior change: An empirical analysis.* New York: John Wiley, 1971.

BORUS, J. F. Neighborhood health centers as providers of primary mental health care. *New England Journal of Medicine.* 1976, *295,* 140.

BORUS, J. F., JANOWITCH, L. A. & KIEFFER, F. The coordination of mental health services at the neighborhood level. *American Journal of Psychiatry,* 1975, *132,* 1177-1181.

CASSEM, N. H., & HACKETT, T. P. Psychiatric consultation in a coronary care unit. *Annals of Internal Medicine,* 1971, *75,* 9.

COLEMAN, J. V. Adaptive integration of psychiatric symptoms in ego regulation. *Archives of General Psychiatry,* 1971, *24,* 17-21.

COLEMAN, J. V. Interdisciplinary implications of primary medical care. Paper presented at the National Interdisciplinary Conference on Primary Health Care, Harriman, New York, 1981.

COLEMAN, J. V., & PATRICK, D. L. Integrating mental health services into primary medical care. *Medical Care,* 1976, *14,* 654-661.

COLEMAN, J. V., & PATRICK, D. L. Psychiatry and general health care. *American Journal of Public Health,* 1978, *68,* 451-457.

COLEMAN, J. V., PATRICK, D. L., & BAKER, S. M. The mental health of children in an HMO program. *Pediatrics,* 1977, *91,* 150-153.

CORNEY, R. The extent of mental and physical ill-health of clients referred to social workers in a local authority department and a general attachment scheme. *Psychological Medicine,* 1979, *9,* 585-589.

CROMBIE, D. L. A model of the medical care system: A general systems approach. In M. M. Hauser (Ed.), The economics of medical care. London: Allen & Unwin, 1972.

CROWELL, E. Redistributive aspects of psychotherapy's inclusion in national health insurance: A summary. *American Psychologist,* 1977, *32,* 731-737.

CUMMINGS, N. A. The anatomy of psychotherapy under national health insurance. *American Psychologist,* 1977, *32,* 711-718.

DHEW. *Inclusion of mental health services in health maintenance organizations: A review of supplemental benefits.* Washington, DC: Author, 1974.

DHEW. *Guidelines for CMHC/CHC linkage grants.* Washington, DC: Author, 1977.

DHEW. *Health, United States, 1978.* Hyatsville, MD: Author, 1978.

DINGWELL, R. Problems of team work in primary care. In S. Lonsdale et al. (Eds.), *Teamwork in the personal social services and health care: British and American perspectives.* Syracuse, NY: Syracuse University School of Social Work, 1980.

ENGEL, G. L. The clinical application of the biopsychosocial model. *American Journal of Psychiatry,* 1980, *137,* 535-543.

ERNST, K. *Die Prognose der Neurosen.* Berlin: Springer, 1959.

GARFIELD, S. R. The delivery of medical care. *Scientific American,* 1970, *222,* 15-23.

GOLDBERG, D. Training family physicians in mental health skill: Implications of recent research findings. In *Mental health services in general health care,* Vol. I. Washington, DC: National Academy of Sciences, 1979.

GOLDBERG, D., KAY, L., & THOMPSON, C. Psychiatric morbidity in general practice and the community. *Psychosomatic Medicine,* 1969, *6,* 565-569.

GOLDBERG, I. D., KRANTZ, G., & LOCKE, B. Z. Effect of a short-term outpatient psychiatric therapy benefit on the utilization of medical services in prepaid group practice medical program. *Medical Care,* 1970, *8,* 419.

GOLDENSOHN, S. S. A prepaid group-practice mental health service as part of a health maintenance organization. *American Journal of Orthopsychiatry,* 1972, *42,* 154-158.

GREENHILL, M. H. The development of liaison programs. In G. Usdin (Ed.), *Psychiatric medicine.* New York: Brunner/Mazel, 1977.

Group for the Advancement of Psychiatry. *Mental health & primary medical care.* Committee on Preventive Psychiatry, 1980.

HOEPER, E. W. Observations on the impact of psychiatric disorder upon primary medical care. In *Mental health services in general health care,* Vol. I Washington, DC: National Academy of Sciences, 1979.

JACOBSON, A. M., REGIER, D. A., & BURNS, B. J. Factors relating to the use of mental health services in a neighborhood health center. *Public Health Reports,* 1978, *93,* 232-239.

JOHNSTONE, A., & GOLDBERG, D. Psychiatric screening in general practice. *Lancet,* 1976, 605-608.

KIESLER, F. Is this psychiatry? In S. E. Goldstein (Ed.), *Concepts of community psychiatry.* Washington, DC: National Institute of Mental Health, 1975.

LEWIS, A. *The state of psychiatry: Essays & addresses.* New York: Science House, 1967.

LIPOWSKI, Z. J. Consultation-liaison psychiatry: An overview. *American Journal of Psychiatry,* 1974, *131,* 623-630.

LIPOWSKI, Z. J. Sensory and information overload: Behavioral effects. *Comprehensive Psychiatry,* 1979, *16,* 199-211.

LOCKE, B. Z., KRANTZ, G., & KRAMER, M. Psychiatric need and demand in a prepaid group practice program. *American Journal of Public Health,* 1966, *56,* 895.

McSWEENEY, A. J. Including psychotherapy in national health insurance: Insurance guidelines and other proposed solutions. *American Psychologist,* 1977, *32,* 722-730.

MORRILL, R. G. Integration of mental health and comprehensive health services in a neighborhood health center. In L. B. Macht et al. (Eds.), *Neighborhood psychiatry.* Lexington, MA: Lexington Books, 1977.

National Academy of Sciences. *A manpower policy for primary care: Report of a study*. Washington, DC: Author, 1978.

NEWHOUSE, J. P., PHELPS, C. E., & SCHWARTZ, W. B. Polity options and the impact of national health insurance. *New England Journal of Medicine,* 1974, *290,* 1345-1359.

PAKULA, L. Mental health in a fee-for-service pediatric practice. In *Mental health services in general health care,* Vol. I. Washington, DC: National Academy of Sciences, 1979.

PATRICK, D. L., EAGLE, J., & COLEMAN, J. V. Primary care treatment of emotional problems in an HMO. *Medical Care,* 1978, *16,* 47-60.

PATRICK, D. L., COLEMAN, J. V., EAGLE, J., & NELSON, E. Chronic emotional problem patients and their families in an HMO. *Inquiry,* 1978, *15,* 166-180.

PATTERSON, D. T. Psychiatric practice in an HMO. *Psychiatric Opinion,* 1976, *13,* 27-31.

PINCUS, H. A. Linking general health and mental health systems of care: Conceptual models of implementations. *American Journal of Psychiatry,* 1980, *137,* 315-320.

The President's Commission on mental health. Executive Order No. 11973, February 17, 1977.

REGIER, D. A., GOLDBERG, I. D., & TAUBE, C. A. The de facto US mental health services system. *Archives of General Psychiatry,* 1978, *35,* 685-693.

RICHMAN, A., & BROWN, M. G. Reimbursement by medicare for mental health services by general practitioners–clinical, epidemiologic and cost containment implications of the Canadian experience. In *Mental health services in general health care,* Vol. I. Washington, DC: National Academy of Sciences, 1979.

RITTLEMEYER, L. E. Continuing education in psychiatry for physicians: Report of a four-year experience. *Journal of the American Medical Association,* 1972, *220,* 710-714.

RITTLEMEYER, L. E., & FLYNN, W. E. Psychiatric consultation in an HMO: A model for education in primary care. *American Journal of Psychiatry,* 1978, *135,* 1089-1093.

SACK, P. G. The stigma of psychiatric referral. *Psychiatric Annals,* 1981, *11,* 33-35.

SCHNIEWIND, H. E. A psychiatrist's experience in a primary care setting. *International Journal of Psychiatry in Medicine,* 1977, *7,* 229-241.

SHEPHERD, M. General practice, mental illness and the British National Health Service. *American Journal of Public Health,* 1979, *64,* 230-232.

SHEPHERD, M., COOPER, B., BROWN, A. C., & KALTON, G. W. *Psychiatric illness in general practice.* London: Oxford University Press, 1966.

SHEPHERD, M., HARWIN, B. G., DEPLA, G., & CAIRNS, V. Social work and the primary care of mental disorder. *Psychological Medicine,* 1979, *9,* 661-669.

SHORTELL, S. M., & DANIELS, R. S. Referral relationships between internists and psychiatrists in fee-for-service practice: An empirical examination. *Medical Care,* 1974, *12,* 229.

SLABY, A. E., POTTASH, A.L.C., & BLACK, H. R. Utilization of psychiatry in a primary care center. *Journal of Medical Education,* 1978, *53,* 752-758.

STRATAS, N. E., and CATHELL, J. L. Psychiatric consultation with community physicians. *Hospital & Community Psychiatry,* 1966, *17,* 26-28.

TESSLER, R., MECHANIC, D., & DIAMOND, M. The effect of psychological distress on physician utilization. *Journal of Health & Social Behavior,* 1976, *17,* 353-364.

WALSH, D. D., & BICKNELL, W. J. Perspectives on neighborhood health centers. In L. Macht et al. (Eds.), *Neighborhood psychiatry.* D.C. Heath & Co., New York, 1977, p. 44.

WATSON, J. H. Differences between physically-minded and psychologically-minded medical practitioners. *British Journal of Psychiatry,* 1966, *112,* 1097-1102.

WATTS, C.A.H. *Depressive disorders in the community.* Bristol: John Wright, 1966.

WEINERMAN, R. E. Report of a study. In MacColl, W. A. *Group practice & prepayment of medical care.* Washington, DC: Public Affairs Press, 1966.

Chapter 13

THE DEINSTITUTIONALIZATION MOVEMENT

ERNEST GRUENBERG

This volume deals with the interaction between the mental health movement and the public health movement. A good approach to understanding the interaction between these two movements is to look at each of them in terms of what has been desired from the other. What are the attractions for interaction? Why did mental health people expect to get anything from public health? Why did public health expect to get anything from mental health?

The theme of this chapter is that each was trying to compensate for internal weaknesses through an alliance that could not compensate for those weaknesses. This chapter focuses on the deinstitutionalization movement as an illustration of this principle. "Deinstitutionalization" is a recent term. It was first used in 1975 by Bertram Brown, Director of the National Institute of Mental Health, who defined it in terms of three essential components:

(1) the prevention of inappropriate mental hospital admissions through the provision of community alternatives for treatment;
(2) the release to the community of all institutional patients who have been given adequate preparation for such change; and

(3) the establishment and maintenance of community support systems for noninstitutionalized persons receiving mental health services in the community.

It is thus a self-righteous label for a wide variety of activities. Much of the printed literature on the subject approaches the issues in terms of ideologies and concepts and/or exercises in rhetorical exegesis. Rose's article and much of the subsequent discussion in a special number of *Health and Society* illustrate this principle.

A practical approach to understanding what this is all about starts with the assumption that the mental health movement is based on the existence of mental disorders among the people of a community. It is a response to the existence of these disorders. There are several things a society can do about the existence of mental disorders among its populance: It can pretend they don't exist; it can provide care and shelter; it can raise some mentally disordered people into exalted roles; it can place them in dependent relationships to the community, depriving them of some of the privileges of the society and assign them various sick roles; it can try to cure them; and it can try to prevent these cases of disorder from occurring.

The mental hygiene movement stems from the last two efforts. Treatment of the mentally ill in mental hospitals was not as good as it should have been at the beginning of this century. Clifford Beers, an ex-patient, wrote a book, *A Mind That Found Itself,* which led to the founding of the mental hygiene movement. From the start, this movement was associated with the public health movement. It was also associated with the social reform movement of the first part of this century. The movement began by concentrating on improving the care of the mentally ill who required hospital care and later became a staunch supporter of mental hospital developments, helping to defend budgets and to raise personnel standards in our mental hospitals. Very early in its development, it became interested in the prevention of mental disorders. "Prevention" was erroneously linked to the Parent Education and Child Guidance Movement and the Public Education Movements.

There was a general belief that mental disorders had their origins early in childhood and that good family environments and good public education, with some guidance from experts in child development, would reduce the frequency of adult mental disorders. The error was to avoid empirical data. These services have not lowered the frequency of mental disorders (see Lemkau, Chapter 1, this volume). This was in a period when both the mental hygiene movement and the public health movement were closely allied with the general reform movement.

THE SOVEREIGN STATES

As noted in the chapters by Lemkau and by Wagenfeld and Jacobs, the development of mental hospitals for the care and treatment of people with mental disorders began in the middle of the 19th century. It reflected a surge in the power of state governments to improve community life and to take on social responsibilities. It was a reform movement that had its origins in the French Revolution and that was reflected in the humanist notion that people with mental disorders were suffering from acute episodes of disorganization of brain functioning and deserved considerate and respectful care. Provided with that, they would recover rapidly. This idea was in opposition to the notion that the mentally ill were permanently impaired individuals who were a burden on the community and who should be given the minimum of necessary care at the local government level.

Mental hospital reform in this country and in Europe was associated with a remarkable woman from Massachusetts who was the spokesperson for the mental hospital movement for three decades in a single-minded and remarkably effective way. Dorothea L. Dix was the true spark of the mental hospital movement. She appealed to the sense of decency by exposing the terrible conditions under which mentally ill people were cared for in jails, poorhouses, and workhouses operated by local governments. She appealed to the state legislatures' sense of growing power and ability to make great changes by urging them to create hospitals that would provide acute treatment under ideal conditions and return the disordered citizen quickly to home, community, and work.

It is important to underline these two elements of the appeal. First, one must say someone else is doing it badly. Second, one must say that we can do it with wonderful, positive effects, usually a net savings in costs. These two elements underline almost every major trend in the mental health movement. In the middle of the last century, local government was the enemy; state government the savior. A sounder approach would have been to define disease as the people's enemy and government as the people's protector.

In summary, the promise of rapid turn-over and return to the community was kept, by and large, in the first decades of the mental hospitals. They were, indeed, acute treatment centers. But some proportion of their admissions never returned successfully to the community. As time went on, a "silting up" of long-term, chronic, severely disabled patients began to fill a larger and larger proportion of the hospital beds. Therapeutic optimism was replaced with therapeutic pessimism. By the time of World War I, a widespread belief had developed that people admitted to mental hospitals hardly ever left, except when they died. This stereotype never really corresponded to reality.

Mental hospital directors were always showing in their annual reports that a very significant proportion of their new admissions were released in a few months, some never to be heard from again. But since the proportion of beds occupied by long-stay patients had come to dominate the organization of the institution, these short-term patients came to be a minor aspect of life in the institution and a minor aspect of the community's perception of what the mental hospital was for. The bulk of the patients, the bulk of the budget, and the bulk of the personnel were involved in long-term institutional care. These mental hospitals became fairly stable communities. They employed the bulk of the psychiatrists in the country, as well as the clinical psychologists and social workers working with the mentally ill. They were the place in which the next generation of professional workers was trained. The leading mental hospital personnel were the leading psychiatric professionals, and they dominated the American Psychiatric Association until the 1950s. The American Psychiatric Association is a later name for the organization founded in 1843 called "The Association of Superintendents of Hospitals for the Insane."

COMMUNITY PSYCHIATRY

Community psychiatry began developing after World War I and was associated with a growth in university medical school departments of psychiatry, on a small level, and the vast development of voluntary agencies running outpatient clinics, mostly for children, and engaged in community education regarding the salubrious development of mental life.

World War II signaled a complete transformation of the power relationships between growing community psychiatry services and the mental hospital services. The armed forces brought in leading psychiatrists from the community psychiatry movement, to a large extent, and mental health services permeated the armed forces in most countries during World War II in a previously unimaginable way. By the end of the war there was widespread recognition that many young people had been found to be unfit for military duty because of mental disorders and that many men had been discharged from the armed forces because of mental disorders contracted during service.

A lesson should have been learned that was not learned. Never before had such a large proportion of potential draftees been rejected because of psychiatric diagnoses in an effort to preserve the armed forces from mental disorders, but never before had such a large proportion of the armed forces been found to be inadequate for military service because of mental disorders. The idea that psychiatrists knew how to screen and select people at low risk for mental disorders so as to produce a low occurrence rate should have died from this experiment. But it didn't. On the contrary, the effort to screen and predict grew, and the effort to diagnose and dispose of also grew.

THE NATIONAL INSTITUTE OF MENTAL HEALTH

Up until the immediate postwar period, the U.S. Public Health Service had had extremely marginal relationships to the mental health movement. In fact, there were only a small number of people for whom the federal government had any responsibility when they became mentally ill. They included merchant seamen, residents of the District of Columbia, Indian reservation residents, and 10-12 rare types of legal and social status in the American population. But for the bulk of American citizens, there is nothing in the Constitution that gives the federal government any responsibility for the mental health of individuals. This was a responsibility of the states. But the states had not played the role, permitting local governments to deal with it as best they could.

Under pressure from the mental hospital reform movement, led by Dorothea L. Dix, the states finally removed the privilege from local governments because they were too corrupt and incapable of doing an effective job. The federal government had been completely left out of such matters. In 1947, when the National Institutes of Health were founded, along with the National Institute of Mental Health, this new entity moved into a situation where there had been no direct accountability or responsibility for the federal government's behavior. This represented a new variety of money in this situation. Almost all government tax money spent on mental health problems up until that time had been at the state level.

The federal appropriations, although not enormously large, had enormous effects on the atmosphere and the direction in which service pattern developments occurred. One package of money was called "community services money," and it went, via the states, to local community services. When the states administered these funds, they were dealing with a small fraction of a percentage of the total state funds available for psychiatric services. However, this tiny amount could only be spent on nonhospital services for people who were not mental hospital patients. The existing services in the community were mainly supported by voluntary agencies that raised their money from community chests.

These small increments in the state budget were significant increments to the total community services budgets through the voluntary agencies. Consequently, they began to grow. The demand for such services and for their development was already present in the communities. Most of the pressure was for child guidance clinics. The leadership of the local mental health associations was demanding more and more community services of this type and not of general purpose outpatient clinics. Even then, much of the rhetoric pointed out that if these expanded, the need for state hospitals would decline.

THE RETURN OF LOCAL GOVERNMENT

These early postwar developments took a sudden, sharp turn in 1954. Local governments had been driven out of the provision of care for the mentally ill by the Dix-Mann reforms of the middle of the 19th century when the mentally ill were made the wards of the state. It became illegal for local jails, poorhouses, and workhouses to contain mentally ill people. This was reversed by a 1954 act of the New York State legislature, called the Community Mental Health Services Act. It authorized local governments to set up mental health agencies within them. These new agencies of local government were authorized to conduct a spectrum of services if the plan had been approved by the relevant state officials in advance. Under those conditions, the state undertook to compensate the local government for 50 percent of the cost of their program. The main emphasis, of course, was on outpatient services, but information and education programs and other services were explicitly specified. These included the following:

(1) community mental health services;
(2) establishment of community mental health boards;
(3) development of preventive, rehabilitative, and treatment services; and
(4) improvement and expansion of existing community services.

It was explicitly recognized at that time by the relevant state officials in the legislature that this was an expansion of the spectrum of care that the local communities wished to initiate for not severely disturbed, mentally disordered individuals. It was not seen as a substitute for mental hospitals. The sponsoring agency for this legislation was the Department of Mental Hygiene, which operated the mental hospitals. Many were uneasy about the tendency for local mental health leaders to think that the mental hospitals could be made unnecessary and fearful that this could undermine the state hospital budgets. It did not have that effect. On the contrary, it made mental health programs more understandable to the legislators, who recognized that the community services were not prepared to take care of the very seriously disturbed individuals who went to the mental hospitals. However, the state officials of the Department of Mental Hygiene, senior psychiatrists who had been brought up in the mental hospitals, were very skeptical about the ability of local governments to provide services at an adequate standard. They were very sensitive on this issue because they had been reared and educated as the state psychiatrists who were repeatedly saving mental patients from mistreatment by local officials. This was not only part of the history they had been taught but part of their everyday experience from working in mental hospitals when they had to inspect jails and poorhouses for the presence of mentally disordered individuals who were not being properly cared for.

The readiness of local governments to use this opportunity was underestimated by everyone involved. Within a few years, over 50 percent of the state's population had local government services under this law. Other states also began to reverse the Dix-Mann formula of the state having a monopoly on the care of the mentally ill and began to authorize local agencies and local governments to become involved again.

IN THE MENTAL HOSPITAL

At the same time, a few mental hospitals had been experimenting with the lessons their directors had learned during World War II. Three British psychiatrists led this change with very little publicity. They had worked in mental hospitals during World War II and felt that they had learned some lessons from the responses to staff shortages. They had found that less-trained staff could take more responsibility. They also found that patients were able to take more responsibility for their own behavior, for one another, and for the management of aspects of hospital life than had been permitted in more conventional mental hospitals. The psychiatrists developed an ideology of delegating responsibility and authority downward to include the patients. They exercised careful discrimination regarding who could be responsible for what. This discrimination was with respect to the individual people, not categories of people. They noticed that everybody took more responsibility in proportion to the extent to which they were given responsibility.

The use of personnel to maintain locked patient care systems had impressed the three psychiatrists as largely wasteful and probably destructive to patients' mental health as well. Consequently, they had begun experimenting with patient care patterns using fewer restrictions on patients and fewer locked wards in their hospitals. By the mid-1950's, three of these hospitals had no locked wards whatsoever. In addition, it was discovered that the release of patients very early in their treatment to return home and continue care with the hospital staff on a day basis or an outpatient basis relieved the hospital of some of its responsibilities and, to their surprise, led to a more speedy recovery. This was called "community care of the severely mentally ill."

For those who were close to these developments, their colleagues' reactions were disturbing. Many of those in public health psychiatry never absorbed the lessons, and American psychiatrists on the whole did not understand what had happened. Those who were not close to what was happening had insufficient background in mental hospital psychiatry to understand what was occurring. Those who had not spent time in mental hospitals had never really accepted the challenge of the clinical and administrative problems that the patients presented. They tended to have a stereotyped notion that mental hospital staff preferred to lock up patients and that they would rather see them sick. They also had a tendency to think that mental hospital staff were poorly trained, poorly educated, and indifferent to the developments in modern psychiatry. Not having accepted the responsibility professionally and personally, it was difficult for them to understand the seriousness of purpose and the conscientiousness with which most mental hospital staff went about their duties. In fact, good mental hospital staff had been trying to find ways of taking care of patients with fewer restrictions and more self-reliance for a long time.

The difficulties of running a comprehensive mental hospital without locked wards are not to be minimized. The combination of legal, clinical, and community responsibilities, which the director of such a hospital must confront, is not at all easy. In fact, to this day only a small proportion of mental hospitals have completely mastered that art. One reason for the difficulty of doing this is the diminished authority of the mental hospital director. This authority has been diminished as much by his colleagues in university departments and state governments as by advocates of patient's rights and the growing infrequency of involuntary certification. It has also been diminished by the inability to recruit main-line American medical school graduates to hospital staff. The ubiquitous general separation of authority from responsibility has played a large part in the failure of mental hospitals and inpatient services in general to master this technique of giving optimum care to the seriously disturbed, mentally ill patient. Because the inpatient experience is the most intensive experience a mentally ill person has with the professional services, if the professionals working in the hospital or other inpatient service are isolated from responsibility before and after the inpatient phase of treatment, nothing but trouble can ensue. The inpatient experience is a central and valuable focus for the organization of long-term treatment plans. This is true of all chronic incurable illnesses, not just of mental disorders.

The startling experiences of those who reorganized the mental hospitals so as to remove the barriers between hospital staff and community services and to make the movement of patients in and out of the mental hospital an extremely fluid phenomenon were lost on American psychiatry in general. The improvement in patient functioning and the reduced frequency with which chronic, severe deterioration in personal and social functioning occurred were quickly extrapolated to the notion that the mental hospital was the cause of such long-term deterioration. While that was true for a small minority of cases, it was not true in general. What the new pattern of care did bring to bear was a greatly enhanced understanding of how to make use of inpatient and outpatient services, as well as other forms of community services that preserved to the maximum the patient's own assets and spontaneous social support systems, and how to gear the community support systems to make the best use of those support systems and assets.

THE PHARMACY TAKES OVER

Meanwhile, in France, a naval surgeon, Laborit, had been developing a drug that was intended to reduce the shock effect of protracted reconstructive surgery by modifying a molecule of some antihistamines to favor the somnerific effect and minimize the antihistamine effect. Chlorpromazine resulted, and Laborit recognized that it would have an effect on mental patients as well. He arranged for a manic seaman, who entered the hospital, to receive treatment with the drug, and it proved to be very effective. The leading French psychiatrists became aware of these developments and started experimenting with their psychiatric patients. They organized an international conference on psychopharmacological agents with target symptoms. These symptoms had never been thought of as susceptible to drug intervention. Sometimes they were called "antipsychotic agents." In general, they did not terminate the disorders but reduced the disturbed and disturbing behavior and thought patterns to less intense levels. These drugs were quickly picked up by American psychiatry and were wrongly regarded as the main cause of all subsequent changes in hospital statistics.

THE LEADERS ARRIVE

American psychiatry's leaders soon began to catch on to the fact that they ought to do something to shape the future. During the year that Kenneth Apple, from Philadelphia, was President-elect, the leadership of the American Psychiatric Association went through a series of private conferences with various people to plan a move to create what later turned out to be the Joint Commission on Mental Health. The commission was created by an act of Congress the subsequent year. At that time, the center of gravity of the leadership of American psychiatry was moving from the alumni of training in state mental hospitals to the alumni of training in university departments of psychiatry. The latter had become numerous and large just after the creation of the NIMH and the availability of clinical training funds for the medical schools. Both groups were strongly represented in the Joint Commission.

The commission's creation represented a major turning point for federal involvement with the public health issue of mentally ill people. But the distance between the public health movement and the mental health movement was symbolized by the fact that the American Public Health Association was not represented on the commission. The day the newspapers announced the existence of the new commission on mental health and mental retardation, the executive board of the American Public Health Association was meeting in New York. They had never heard that such a commission was about to be created. At the same time, a group of public mental health workers was meeting at the airport in Buffalo to discuss what sort of arrangement could be made as a forum for public mental health workers. There was some discussion of creating an affiliated organization that would meet simultaneously with the American Public Health Association. There was also discussion about setting up some mechanism within the American Orthopsychiatric Association, which tended to take a community point of view.

A telephone call came from the Executive Director of the American Public Health Association saying that the executive board felt that the existence of a national commission on some aspect of health that did not include the American Public Health Association showed the need for a mental health section in the American Public Health Association. The board had created such a section and designated a number of us meeting at the Buffalo airport as the first section council to organize the section. One factor that influenced this decision was that the most aggressive section of the American Public Health Association, Medical Care, was rejecting papers dealing with the organization of psychiatric services from a medical care point of view.

Looking back, it becomes obvious that a new section created for the above reasons was not destined for great success. The American Public Health movement, as symbolized by the American Public Health Association, had simply been out of the action *ultimately* with respect to mental health services. The new federal legislation creating the Joint Commission on Mental Retardation and Mental Health was developed without input from the sections of the American Public Health Association that should have been paying attention to mental disorders. Both the mental health workers in the community and the mental hospital leaders recognized that community services were becoming more and more important and that the technology of psychiatric treatment was changing rapidly, leading to less and less emphasis on institutional care. The Joint Commission's perspective can be summarized, in my opinion, by saying that it was oriented toward the increasing role of the mental health professional, particularly the psychiatric profession, and looking toward a larger federal investment in the provision of services.

The outcome was not exactly predictable. The commission's report, which took the form of a volume entitled *Action for Mental Health,* did not recommend very specific things about improved services. It did imply that the mental hospitals should be less voluminous and have fewer patients. It is probably true to say that the report was a disappointment to the leading officials in the federal government who believed that the time was right for getting a larger commitment from Congress for developing services. The unpredictable event that occurred was the election of John Kennedy and his decision that mental retardation would become "his disease" in the way that poliomyelitis had been Franklin D. Roosevelt's. This was thought, apparently, to be good for the image of a leading politician. Much negotiation went on between the NIMH personnel, the American Psychiatric Association leadership, and the White House advisors to the Kennedys. Mental retardation was permitted to include mental health, and in the end, mental health began to precede mental retardation in the ground-breaking presidential message of 1963 and the accompanying legislation.

The failure of the Joint Commission to produce anything that the NIMH could use to strengthen its position mobilized the NIMH for the first time to develop policy statements. Utilizing the publicity surrounding the commission's report as a lever, the NIMH then came forward with something entirely new: the Mental Health Center legislation recommendation embodied in Kennedy's message to Congress. From then on, the leadership and policy formation fell into the hands of the NIMH and the constituencies it created around the University Chairmen of Psychiatry and the leaders of mental health centers.

The Community Mental Health Center was a symbol that was developed to focus attention on the opportunity for federal funds to change rapidly the balance of community versus mental hospital resources. In the testimony in support of this legislation, the National Institute of Mental Health implied that a 50 percent reduction in the mental hospital census would follow within a decade. By 1963 this was a prediction that could be made without too much exaggeration of the trend that had already begun in 1955 of falling hospital censuses (see Figure 13.1). However, the drop was not very dramatic until after the 1966 Amendment to the Social Security Act, which created the federal Medicare and Medicaid programs. Through those programs, elderly people began to be placed in nursing homes in preference to mental hospitals, and the balance shifted over remarkably from mental hospital occupancy rates for the elderly to an epidemic of nursing home construction and nursing home placements. Other age groups also shifted to nursing homes, but not in such a dramatic way. The notion that nursing homes are less "institutional" than mental hospitals is false. The best mental hospitals were far superior to average nursing homes and far less restrictive of personal freedom (see Figure 13.2).

The amendments to the Social Security Act had an even larger impact on the care of mentally ill people than the actions associated with the creation of the mental health centers. While some leaders in public health and psychiatry played an active part in the formulation of the Medicare and Medicade legislation, they had little interest in or understanding of the implications for chronic mental illness here in this country. The impact of these amendments on the financing of state mental hospitals, nursing homes, and mental health centers was not appreciated for a number of years by those responsible for setting policies with respect to those agencies.

THE COMPETITION FOR THE MOST RAPIDLY DROPPING CENSUS OF MENTAL HOSPITAL PATIENTS

In each state mental hospital, directors vied for a better report on a dropping census. The states began to compete with one another for publicity, with one claiming to have dropped its census more than another. A falling mental hospital census became a fetish and an end in itself, without regard for the

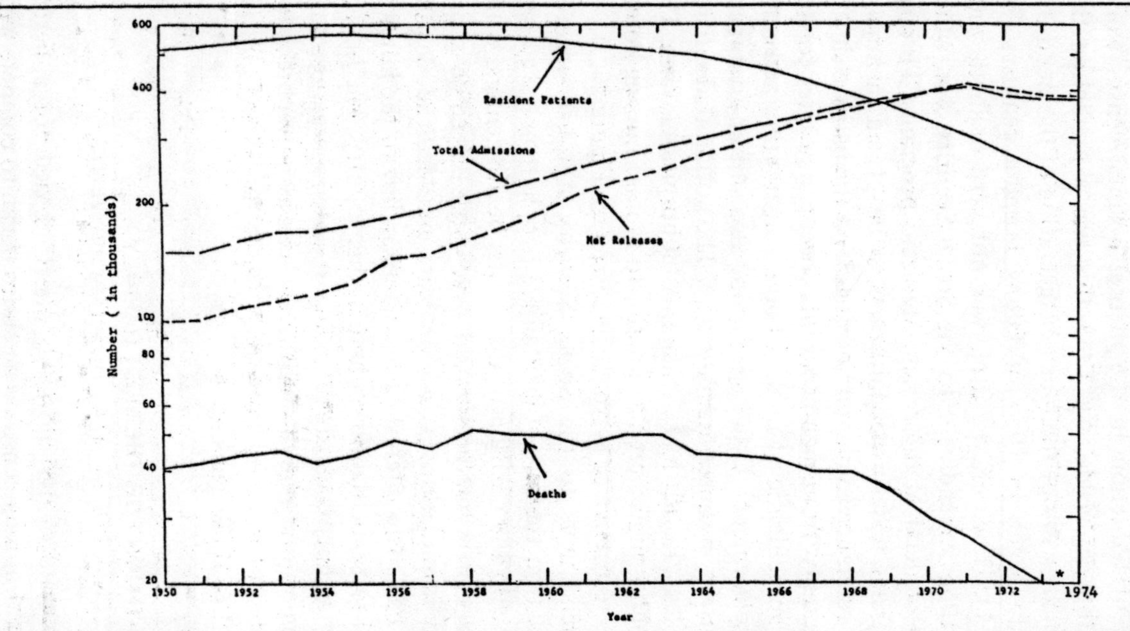

Figure 13.1 Number of Resident Patients, Total Admissions, Net Releases, and Deaths, State and County Mental Hospitals, United States, 1950-1974

*There were 19,899 deaths in 1973 and 16,597 deaths in 1974.

SOURCE: National Institute of Mental Health, **Psychiatric Services and the Changing Institutional Science, 1950-1985**. DEW Publication No. ADM77-433. Washington, DC: Government Printing Office.

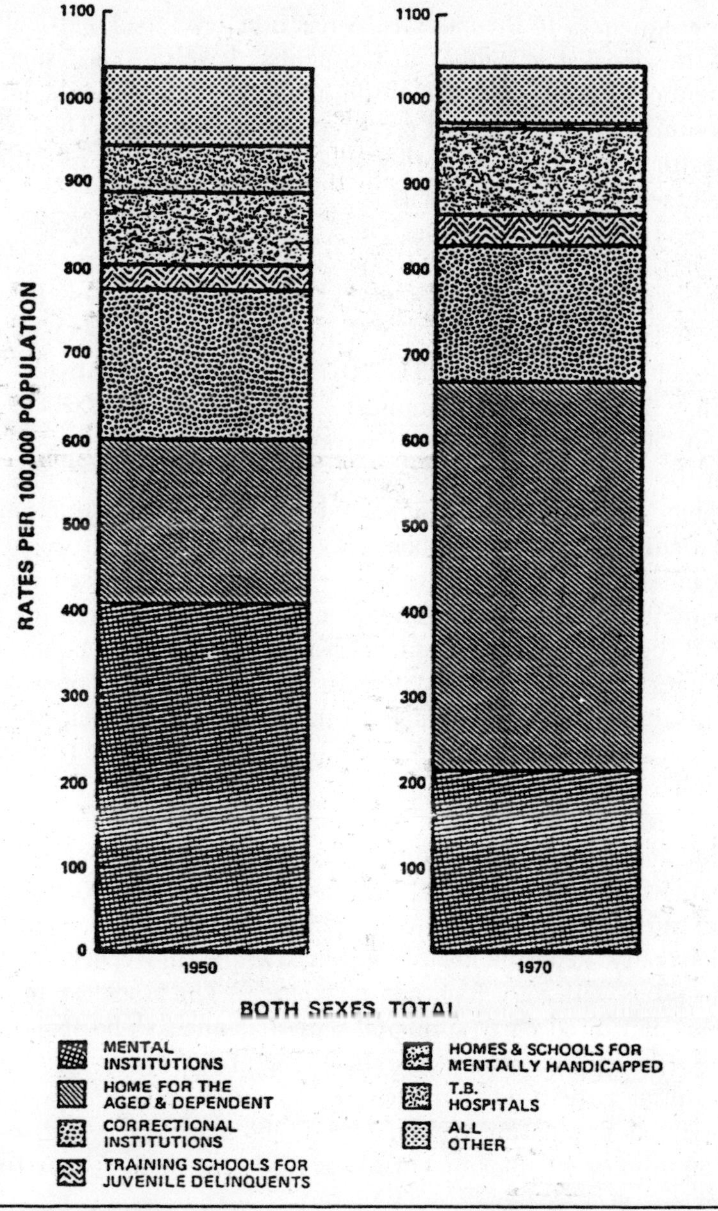

Figure 13.2 Distribution by Persons in Institutions per 100,000 Population by Type of Institution, Both Sexes, United States, 1950 and 1970

SOURCE: National Institute of Mental Health, **Psychiatric Services and the Changing Institutional Scene, 1950-1985.** DEW Publication No. ADM77-433. Washington, DC: Government Printing Office.

consequences to the patients. A reaction developed, particularly in the local government departments of welfare, accusing the mental hospital systems of dumping helpless patients into a community that was not prepared to care for them. The mental health centers played only a trivial role in the care of patients released from such hospitals.

Some excellent investigative reporting was done exposing the fact that some former patients were having devastating experiences due to their incompetence to care for themselves. Bearing such titles as "The Chronic Mentally Ill Shuffle to Oblivion" (Reich and Siegel, 1973), "Discharged Mental Patients–Are They Really in the Community?" (Lamb and Goertzel, 1971), and "The New Snake Pits" (Newsweek, 1978), articles appeared in the professional literature and popular press questioning the value of reforms that appeared to worsen the situation of patients. Such scandals began to outnumber and outweigh the scandals that had always occurred when a released mental patient attacked or killed someone. Mental hospitals in the past had been defensive about releasing patients who committed crimes. Now they were defensive about the neglect of patients but continued to get orders from above to drop their hospital censuses and blame the local communities for failure to provide services.

Pressures developed for local mental health centers to pick up the responsibility for the care of released mental hospital patients. But local mental health centers tend to be dependent on third-party payments for patient care. They are frequently in university departments of psychiatry and university teaching hospitals with very high per-day charges. The homeless, moneyless, uninsured chronic mental patient tended to be abandoned by the community mental health centers. Thus, the mental hospital patient load moved into a more and more seriously disabled population as the less disabled were released to the community whether or not it was ready for them or they for it.

THE RISING PREVALENCE OF INSTITUTIONALIZATION

If the falling mental hospital census was combined with the nursing home census in the United States as a whole, the prevalence of hospitalization or nursing home placement rose during this period. Figure 13.1 shows this rise.

DECLINING RATE OF INCREASE IN FEDERAL APPROPRIATIONS

During the Nixon Administration there was a period of difficulty in gaining support for increased federal spending for both psychiatric and other professional mental health training and for the expansion and development of community mental health centers. It was in this context that the General Accounting Office asked for material on the process of deinstitutionalization and Bertram Brown's policy statement, giving the concept of deinstitutionalization its initial baptism. This was the same context in which leaders were trying to develop a replay of the Joint Commission on Mental Health. Again, a presidential election unexpectedly changed the environment for such a reactivation of something like the Joint Commission.

Jimmy Carter, as Governor of Georgia, with his wife's assistance had made mental disorder "his" illness. Therefore, the creation of his Presidential Commission on Mental Health was a natural wedding of the forces that were trying to give Carter a role for his wife and an image with respect to concerns with one or another category of ill people and those who were seeking to reactivate something like the Joint Commission (The President's Commission, 1978). The commission did draw attention to the problems of mental health, but did not lead to any gross increases in appropriations. It may have slowed the rate of decrease of appropriations, and it may have shifted the center of gravity somewhat toward preventive activities. But it did not lead to any great increase in federal initiatives financially. By that time, the amount of money that came from the federal government to the care of the mentally ill by Medicare and Medicaid far outweighed in dollars the influence the NIMH could muster.

THE ABANDONMENT OF THE SERIOUSLY MENTALLY ILL

The deinstitutionalization policies leading to the dramatic reductions in state mental hospital censuses in the 1970s can be seen as a rapid acceleration of a trend to transfer financial responsibility for the chronically mentally ill patient from the state mental health departments to the social welfare system. The present crisis of abandonment of the seriously mentally ill has arisen because no similar transfer of responsibility for their care and treatment has taken place. The erosion of state mental hospital responsibility has created a situation in which psychiatry's most helpless patients have no recourse against a general tendency of all medical services to reject its most unrewarding patients. While the seriously mentally ill are a visible problem causing much concern, and espousing their cause has become a very gratifying role, the tendency has been to advocate solutions that are someone else's responsibility to execute. Social welfare departments are not equipped to provide the psychiatric attention that many of these patients need on a continuing basis. But such proposals as "remedicalizing psychiatry" and "mainstreaming the chronic mental patient into general medical practice" are simply code phrases for saying that psychiatry and the mental health facilities do not want responsibility for the seriously ill mental patient. Robert Morris (1970) has aptly described this "reject syndrome" as "a phenomenon in which service-providing agencies and families find it unpalatable or undesirable or unacceptable to expend the energy the mentally disabled require; and as a result, each finds a rationalization for trying to reject the giving of attention in the hope that some other organization or entity will assume the responsibility."

The road leading to the demise of state responsibility for the seriously mentally ill and the current crisis of abandonment was paved with all the best intentions. Tragically for the seriously mentally ill, the current policies underlying the pattern of abandonment are based on erroneous interpretations of what patients need and what our current techniques can produce to help people with serious mental disorders. These interpretations have been systematically encouraged by a general crisis in government and social policy. The fashion has been for "cost-benefit" reasoning, dramatic efforts to reduce operating budgets, and the shifting of responsibilities away from one element of government to another. We can identify six errors shared by both the advocates and the opponents of deinstitutionalization.

The first is that a falling mental hospital census necessarily indicates program success. In the early years of the deinstitutionalization movement, a falling hospital census was a reasonable index of progress toward reducing the number of long-term patients. Later, this became a goal in itself, with pressure by policymakers for an even greater reduction in the census.

A second error was the belief that if a falling census was an index of success, a rising readmission rate was evidence of failure. The release into the community of long-term patients required the recognition that many of these persons would require intermittent, short-term crisis readmissions. To do otherwise would be to abandon responsibility for their care.

Some of the early rhetoric of several of the leaders of community mental health argued that hospitalization per se, was harmful to mental patients. While it is true that hospitalization that undermines the patient's ability for self-support is injurious, it is also true that short-term hospitalization can be beneficial in several ways. For example, it can provide a respite for the patient's family and help to avoid rejection of the patient. A short stay in the hospital can also help avoid long-term institutional care by speeding the resolution of crises associated with the disorder. Additional benefits of hospitalization are discussed in Gruenberg (1974).

In a related vein, it has been argued that state hospital care is inherently restrictive. This is not so, since good hospital care can often be provided with far fewer restrictions on the life of the patient than in nursing homes, "welfare" hotels, and locked psychiatric wards in general hospitals.

One of the problems associated with deinstitutionalization has been a lack of continuity and coordination between the state hospital and community treatment teams. The creation of new treatment facilities and new categories of personnel has only exacerbated the problem, particularly for the chronic, seriously mentally ill patients. These patients often require conditional releases, with the kind of close and careful follow-up that is possible only with a unified, clinical-team approach.

The final error has been the argument that a reduction in state hospital beds will automatically result in a cost saving. The experience of several decades of deinstitutionalization indicates the opposite: The decline in patient census has been accompanied by an increase in expenditures for state mental hospitals. The competition between mental health policymakers and budget directors to reduce governmental costs has resulted in patient abandonment, not cost savings.

THE CHRONICALLY MENTALLY ILL AS A NEW PRIORITY

The chronically mentally ill have become a new priority in the last few years because those with a serious disability have been abandoned by the state governments, as indicated earlier. A generation of new chronically mentally ill patients with severe disability has arisen since chronic hospitalization became unavailable in the last 15-20 years. These people are in the community, and they are a burden to community mental health centers and programs. There is a growing interest in seeing what can be done about them.

DEINSTITUTIONALIZATION AS WISHFUL THINKING

The attempt to develop community services in the name of preventing the need for hospital services has come full circle, and its weakness has been exposed by the sequence of events discussed here. Deinstitutionalization is only one extreme manifestation of the notion that the chronically disabled mentally ill are a product of the mental hospital. The most extreme form of this ideology was expressed by Thomas Szasz (1973) in his book, *The Manufacture of Madness.* Szasz has maintained an acceptable position within American Psychiatry, while the leaders of American psychiatry have tried to divorce themselves from his extreme positions at various points. But implicit in many of the deinstitutionalization slogans and actions has been the notion that if the chronic mental hospitals didn't exist, the chronically disabled, helpless patient would not exist. There was never any evidence for this idea, and it is contrary to the realities of our technology. Chronic mental illnesses continue to occur and continue to be incurable by current techniques. Programs for the care of seriously disabled mental patients must be organized and are a responsibility of the society. The profession does not do itself a favor by pretending that this problem could be dealt with by an increase in office psychiatry or university outpatient psychiatry. Meanwhile, the move to "deinstitutionalize" seems to suggest that because the mental hospital censuses are falling, chronic institutionalization is falling in frequency. Figure 13.1 shows this to be a fallacy.

SUMMARY

The public mental health movement has not ended. In its present form it is rather helpless, but there is a higher density of professional mental health workers than ever before in history. There is also a higher density of full-time mental health planners, organizers of policy, and implementers of programs. There are more people being trained in mental health occupations than ever before in history, and there are more techniques for dealing with mental disorders now than ever before in history. And yet there is no coherent sense of direction regarding where the next movement should take us. "Deinstitutionalization" has labeled a decade of incoherent convulsions, both in practice and in the literature, while the prevalence of chronic institutionalization in the presence of mental disorders has been rising. Likewise, the prevalence of mentally impaired individuals is also rising, not falling (Gruenberg, 1977; Kramer, Chapter 5, this volume).

The next focus of service must be on the chronic mentally ill person and the undoing of the fantastic fragmentation of services to such people. "Case managers" cannot undo fragmentation. For the chronically mentally ill, we are not doing as well as we know how.

The focus of research must be on lowering the incidence of chronic mental disorders, particularly those that are increasing in prevalence, since the mortality rate associated with serious mental disorders has been falling due to advancing medical technology.

There is no obvious organizational base for the mental health movement of the future. No single group of professionals is committed to reducing the burden of mental disorders. The NIMH staff is a limited but powerful resource. The American Psychiatric Association is a growing center of gravity, but its seriousness of purpose with respect to the needs of the public will always be questionable because of the economic interests of its membership base. The American Public Health Association is in the midst of a prolonged crisis as its own membership base enlarges each year with more and more peripheral professionals playing a larger and larger role in determining the association's policy. The alliance between social reform and public health still has a sentimental base, but no longer an objective one. Modern public health technology tends to postpone social reform because infectious killing diseases can be controlled even under apalling living conditions. As the Public Health Association grows in size, the safety of the environment worsens. The schools of public health are not a suitable base of leadership either, because they are geared toward feeding the bureaucracies that keep the membership of the American Public Health Association growing. The slowly growing organizations of family members of affected people are the only highly motivated advocates.

At the present time, therefore, there is no obvious organizational base for a public health movement addressed to finding ways to decrease the frequency with which people suffer from mental disorders. That would have been the public health approach of the old days, but it is not the public health approach of today.

References

BACHRACH, L. L. *Deinstitutionalization: An analytic review and sociological perspective.* USDEW Publication No. (ADM) 76-351. Washington, DC: Government Printing Office, C. 1976.

BEERS, C. *A mind that found itself.* New York: Longmans, Green, 1908.

DEUTSCH, A. *The mentally ill in America.* Garden City, NY: Doubleday, 1937.

DEUTSCH, A. *The shame of the states.* New York: Harcourt Brace Jovanovich, 1948.

FELIX, R. Senate committee on Education and Labor, *Hearings* on S. 11600, National Neuropsychiatric Act, 79th Congress, 2nd Session. Washington, DC: Government Printing Office, 1946.

GRUENBERG, E. M. Obstacles to optimal psychiatric service delivery systems. *Psychiatric Quarterly,* 1972, *46*(4), 483-496.

GRUENBERG, E. M. Benefits of short-term hospitalization in *Intervention in schizophrenia: Current development in treatment.* New York: Behavioral, 1974.

GRUENBERG, E. M. The failures of success. *Milbank Memorial Fund Quarterly,* 1977, *55*(1), 3-24.

GRUENBERG, E. M. and ARCHER, J. Abandonment of the seriously mentally ill. *Milbank Memorial Fund Quarterly,* 1979, *79,* 485-506.

GRUENBERG, E. M. and BELLIN, S. S. The impact of mental disease on society, in A. M. Clausen et al. (eds.), *Explorations in social psychiatry.* New York: Basic Books, 1957.

GRUENBERG, E. M. and KOLB, L. C. The Washington Heights Continuous Care Project, in L. C. Kolb et al. (eds.), *Urban challenges to psychiatry: The case history of a response.* Boston: Little, Brown, 1969.

Joint Commission on Mental Illness and Health. *Action for mental health.* New York: Basic Books, 1961.

KENNEDY, J. F. *Message relative to mental illness and mental retardation, February 5.* 88th Congress, Doc. No. 58. Washington, DC: Government Printing Office, 1963.

LAMB, H. and GOERTZEL, V. Discharged mental patients–are they really in the community? *Archives of General Psychiatry,* 1971, *24,* 29-34.

Milbank Memorial Fund. Reports on group visits to Great Britain's community based open mental hospitals, in *Steps in the development of integrated psychiatric services.* New York: Milbank Memorial Fund, 1960.

MORRIS, J. N. *The uses of epidemiology* (2nd ed.). London: Livingston, 1970.

New York State Department of Mental Hygiene. Community Mental Health Service Act, Article 8-A in the *Mental hygiene law and general orders.* Utica, New York, 1954.

Newsweek. The new snake pits. 1978, May 15, 93-94.

The President's Commission on Mental Health. *Report to the President,* Vol. 1. Washington, DC: Government Printing Office, 1978.

REICH, R. and SIEGEL, L. Psychiatry under seige: The chronically mentally ill shuffle to oblivion. *Psychiatric Annals,* 1973, *3,* 35-55.

ROSE, S. Deciphering deinstitutionalization. *Milbank Memorial Fund Quarterly,* 1979, *57,* 430-455.

SWAZEY, J. P. *Chlorpromazine in psychiatry: A study of therapeutic innovation.* Cambridge, MA: MIT Press, 1974.

SZASZ, T. *The manufacture of madness: A comparative study of the inquisition and the mental health movement.* Paladin: Frogmore, St. Albans, Herts, 1973.

WOODWARD, L. E. The mental hygiene movement–more recent developments, in C. Beers, *A mind that found itself.* New York: Doubleday, 1948.

Chapter 14

REFLECTIONS FROM THE 21st CENTURY

ALAN D. MILLER

I ask you to imagine yourself in the year 2000 and to consider our professional preoccupations at that time.

Twenty years. Not a very long time. All of us can find some order in our recollections of the last twenty years, but consider for a moment how difficult it would have been to predict them. There were in 1960 some extrapolations that we could have made to 1980. We could see an accelerating discrepancy between the world's population and the world's resources and an increase in the percentage of the world's population whose survival was in danger. But much of what has become an important part of the texture of all of our lives would have been unintelligible.

Here is a list of ten words or phrases that would have been unintelligible in 1960:

(1) Kennedy and King
(2) Medicaid
(3) the Pill
(4) the Beatles
(5) *Silent Spring*
(6) Vietnam
(7) tricyclic drugs
(8) the Six-Day War

(9) Gay Rights
(10) OPEC

With this brief exercise in humility and retrospection (and there are many other lists we could have made), the reader will be, I hope, more forgiving in judging my forecast.

Yes, we in the mental health profession will still be meeting in October of the year 2000, and that is my most optimistic prediction. We have survived. We are still working together, trying to solve problems, exchanging ideas, arguing, comforting each other in the face of our shortcomings.

We are still the mental health group, the most assorted in the association, our margins still blurred. The association itself has changed. No more APHA. We are a part of the World Health Association. The meeting is being held in Mexico City, which has just become the most populous metropolitan area in the world–slightly larger than São Paolo in Brazil. There are fifteen simultaneous meetings being held around the world and many smaller, local meetings, all joined electronically with both sight and sound. All the proceedings are instantly translated into the six official languages: Chinese, Spanish, English, Swahili, Hindi, and Russian. This year, for the first time, a new, seventh, transnational language is being used experimentally. We are at the North American regional meeting in Detroit, which is a major distribution point for four-wheeled, solar-powered vehicles. (And that is my last excursion into science fiction.)

THE PROGRAM

(A) A Symposium on Long-Term Epidemiologic Studies

1. The distribution of retarded mental development associated with starvation during the first five years of life;
2. The declining prevalence of chronic depressive reactions accompanying the successful control of schistosomiasis; which, at its peak, had a world prevalence of 220 million;
3. The incidence of mental disorders among octogenarians, a ten-year case register study comparing Rochester, New York, USA, Lagos, Nigeria, and Tientsin, China.

(B) A Conference on Social Support Systems for People with Schizophrenia

1. *The Town That Found Itself,* a report of a community self-help project in Forest Hills, New York, USA;
2. World Bank financing of a multinational Social Security system for the chronically disabled;
3. Vulnerability as part of the human condition: a health insurance plan in Cuba, in which premiums and benefits are paid in service units.

(C) A Round Table on the Education of Health Personnel

1. Specialization and its antidotes;
2. Training for nurturance, long-term care, and rehabilitation;
3. Epidemiology as a basic health science.

(D) Psychological Implications of Social Change

1. Incentives and stresses in family size reduction in Sri Lanka;
2. Artistic expression in communal societies—is it at risk?
3. Time and space perspectives: converting the supremacy illusion to cooperative self-interest.

(E) An annual endowed lecture always on the same subject, "The Failures of our Success," sometimes called the Gruenberg Lecture, because Ernest Gruenberg had used the phrase in 1977 to describe growing problems of long-term chronic illness created by our success in thwarting their fatal complications. Since a consideration of this ancient and inexorable phenomenon is always timely and important, the World Health Organization co-sponsors this event with our section.

Thus ends the program.

This program, as I tried to imagine it, kept getting out of hand, and it may strike many as rarefied, imprecise, and self-indulgent. It is all of those things, even though it was intended to be quite the reverse. When I set out on this exploration, I found myself losing landmarks, moving too quickly from observation to speculation to abstraction; from clear paths to wide zones to trackless spaces, and I needed something to keep me in touch, force me to focus, comfort me. In the process, I found myself sorting out several themes, intermingled but still traceable, and these in turn began to shape the October 2000 meeting in my mind. Then the program began to take on a life of its own. I can now step back from it and find those themes expressed, along with some surprises. What are the themes?

Interdependence—the world as an organism in which there are no isolated events. We have always known it and yet have found it almost impossible to live by, and that is a paradox which we can no longer afford. The consequences of interdependence intrude palpably in our daily lives. Connections so constant and so close to the surface that we can pick them up and identify them any time we choose. The time between connected events grows shorter and shorter, as has the time for us to become aware of them. Rainfall in China affects schooling plans in an Iowa wheat-growing household. Family size in Japan affects the reaction to a community residence for mentally ill adults in Detroit. The bombing of a synagogue in Paris upsets a medical school class in Portland, Oregon, the next day. A squirt of fluorocarbon in Oslo affects the ozone layer everywhere. Preston Cloud (1978), head of the School of Earth Sciences at the University of Minnesota, writes: "The air mixes so pervasively and constantly that virtually every breath you take contains some atoms exhaled by every other person who has ever lived, by Abraham, by Confucius, by Cleopatra, by Ghengis Khan."

But such abstractions are for editorial writers, sermonizers, college rap sessions. We actually live and know how to live in much smaller places, e.g., our skins, our families. Sometimes we can extend ourselves to our neighborhoods, even from time to time to our national borders. Is it at least possible for us to enlarge the perspective within which we live our circumscribed lives? Can we find ways to consider both figure and ground, to sense without panic, perhaps even with a feeling of enlarged capacity, that we are also indissolubly linked?

As we stretch the limits of our imagination, we discover another reason for pulling back—a heightened sense of discrepancy. We are all linked in a pattern of awesome inequities. And those of us in the best position to comprehend these inequities and perhaps to act also appear to have the most to lose by changing this state of affairs. Who are we to poke around where even bankers fear to tread? Robert McNamara could not complete his valedictory address to the World Bank because he was so moved by the high tragedy and personal griefs inevitable unless we can redistribute the world's goods. The headline in the September 1980 issue of "The Nation's Health" reads: "The World 2000–crowded, unhealthy." The issue predicts a world "more crowded, less stable ecologically, and more vulnerable to disruption . . . 1.3 billion malnourished people." All of this unless there are "long-term solutions, depending on numerous nations around the world" (Cloud, 1980).

Do we in mental health, on a more limited but no less important scale, have analogous problems of redistribution? Consider the people with long-term illnesses and, in particular, one of the long-term mental illnesses. As more and more of them have continued to live more and more of their lives outside of an all-purpose, man-made environment, taking their chances with the rest, many have continued to require a greater measure of support, both physical and emotional, than do those in good health. Such support is not an act of charity but a simple acknowledgment of mutual responsibilities and a joined fate. Can we think up ways to make vivid and particular the common benefits, the self-interest, served by supporting the vulnerable who turn out eventually to be all of us? Do we have the imagination and discipline to design steps in that direction that are within our capacities?

We can look even closer to home. How do we in the health profession distribute our energies? How do we decide what to learn, what to study, in what places to work, with whom, to what end? Each practitioner, each profession, has always had to come to terms with problems beyond its scope, questions beyond its knowledge, tasks larger than its capacities. "Life is short and the art is long," said Hippocrates. Each group and each period has had to subdivide the work, to specialize. Herodotus, writing in the 5th century, B.C., described the practice of medicine in Egypt: It is divided in many branches, so that each physician treats one disease and no more. Therefore, physicians abound, some for the eyes, some for the head, some for the teeth, some for the belly, and some for obscure ailments."

Specialization in itself is neither new, nor avoidable, nor pernicious. Its characteristic problems are that it may serve its practitioners more than its beneficiaries, that it requires constant regrouping, that it loses sight of wholes, and that it is self-enhancing. We get better at what we do, and we tend to do what we are better at.

Consider the education of medical students in the United States in 1980. This talented, socially responsible, privileged group of women and men are taught the sciences and arts of acute intervention, practiced in a controlled setting with high technology and solitary decision making. They learn to deal with crises. Well and good, and very demanding. But it is not enough. They tend to unlearn perspective, the human and social context, and often why they came to medical school. We are also increasingly neglecting some important problems, and in so doing shrinking in public support, public esteem, and self-esteem. As our students sort themselves out, shape their careers, and choose specialties, they do not consider—because they are neither aware of the choices nor educated to pursue them—the care and study of the chronically ill and the elderly, rehabilitation, health education, community medicine, or simply how to be the health counselor for individuals and families throughout their lives in health and illness.

I both overstate and omit, but I don't invent. There are important parts of our responsibilities as health professionals which we are neglecting, and the neglect has been self-enhancing. I speak of medical students because they are the group with whom I now spend most of my time, and I am devoted to them. I think the problem applies to all health professionals, however.

The professional requirements for working with patients having long-term mental illnesses are difficult. The techniques are subtle, changes often slow, successes modest, the variables many and often outside our control. Yet we must find ways to bring the talents of our teachers and our students to these problems so that the work will be immediately less lonely and so it will begin to be more fruitful. The health professions must, like all the rest, reexpand their limits, once again to include all of its constituents.

Working with people who have a chronic mental illness is a consequence of our earlier successes in treating their acute phases, which doesn't diminish those successes. Our crowded planet is also a result of earlier successes. Every moment can blame its predecessors. But the generations of change are getting shorter, and it seems as if we are running out of time.

As a species, we have not been very good at anticipation. Planning ahead is something we only do in retrospect, and our ineptness has made us both laugh and cry. We don't have time to evolve biologically into a more foresighted creature. Are we capable of a kind of social evolution? Are we capable of learning in time that the strengths of any of us are undermined by the weaknesses in all of us, that the education of one person does not build upon the ignorance of another but on the education of others? That the health of one does not depend on the illness of others? That the safety of one cannot be built on danger to others? We need measures of general well-being that go beyond GNP. Preston Cloud (1978) suggests an EHC quotient–Enhancement of the Human Condition–and he suggests that we might use as a starter the PQL (Physical Quality of Life) index developed by the Overseas Developmental Council in Washington, D.C. In this index, equal weight is given to literacy, infant mortality, and life expectancy.

I have, in looking ahead, meandered back and forth between being there in the year 2000 and getting there. I don't know even now whether I have been looking in the right direction. Still, one needs an article of faith to live by as one searches. I might suggest the following from the writer, Frank Hercules: "The blessings of history are often bestowed in impenetrable disguises."

References

CLOUD, P. *Cosmos, earth, and man.* New Haven, CT: Yale University Press, 1978.

CLOUD, P. *The Nation's Health,* September 1980.

GRUENBERG, E. M. The failures of success. *Millbank Memorial Fund Quarterly,* 1977, *55*(1), 3-24.

HERODOTUS. *History.* Book II, Chapter 84.

Part VI

SUMMARY AND EPILOGUE

Chapter 15

FUTURE DIRECTIONS IN PUBLIC MENTAL HEALTH

MORTON O. WAGENFELD
PAUL V. LEMKAU
BLAIR JUSTICE

Commemorating the anniversary of the Mental Health Section of the American Public Health Association was the spur for considering some of the salient issues in both the past and future of public mental health. The chapters in this book have attempted to bring them together. Using these chapters as a framework, we will attempt a synthesis and a projection of our vision of the future. In some respects, writing in early 1982, with the full impact of "Reaganomics" being felt, our thoughts may be more pessimistic than the views of some of the contributors whose chapters were written earlier.

In different ways, the chapters in this book have dealt with the sociopolitical climate and the major issues in service delivery that existed in 1955. Briefly, the state hospital census had reached its peak. As a system of care, its inadequacies had been widely publicized. The experiences of military psychiatry in World War II had demonstrated the efficacy of newer modes of treatment, as well as uncovering large numbers of previously undetected cases of disorder. The community roots of mental disorder and the possibility of its treatment there were beginning to be explored and articulated widely. Attention to the community roots of disorder also helped to broaden the narrow Freudian focus on the primacy of family dynamics to include sociocultural and political factors in the concept of etiology. The NIMH began to emerge as a force for stimulating and supporting training, research, and service delivery. The Mental Health Study Act, the work of the Joint Commission (1961), and an increasingly active and articulate alliance of professional and lay groups in the mental health field helped create an increased awareness of the problems of mental disorder. Psychoactive medications, which made feasible the release of patients from custodial institutions, were beginning their development during this period. Finally, the development of Medicare and Medicaid also made it possible to pay for the support of patients outside of a mental hospital.

With these forces as context, the growth of public mental health in the past 25 years has been remarkable. The "CMHC era" has significantly altered the mental health delivery system in a number of ways. The over 700 CMHCs in operation today represent a new mode of service delivery. The locus of care shifted from the state hospital to the community, and populations previously underserved or not served at all were brought into treatment. The rapid growth and development of CMHCs also created demands for more persons trained in the core mental disciplines, as well as for new kinds of care-givers—the new professionals, or paraprofessionals. The optimism surrounding the birth of CMHCs also gave rise to renewed optimism about the possibility of preventing mental disorder. Changes in the types and strategy of service delivery have also come about as a result of the CMHC movement. Finally, the CMHC represented a significant new role for the federal government in the alleviation of stress and disorder.

In no less significant a fashion, psychiatric epidemiology has undergone change. In keeping with an accelerating focus on the community roots of disorder, there was a substantial shift in the conceptual and methodological basis of the field. During the early part of the period, when state hospitals were the major locus of care for the seriously ill, emphasis was on the measurement of hospital admissions. As a result, estimates of the prevalence of disorder were quite low. Later, with an increasing interest in the community, attention turned toward estimating diagnosed or treated prevalence. In the early 1960s, interest shifted toward global measures of impairment and an attempt to derive estimates of true prevalence. These were, of course, considerably higher than those obtained from the previous approaches. Currently, in the attempt to estimate true prevalence, there is an attempt to meld clinical and epidemiological concerns with instruments that can better serve the needs of both groups in the planning of services. These changes have created challenges and opportunities for researchers and planners.

Just as the developments of the past 25 years—especially CMHCs—had to be considered in the context of the ameliorative optimism of the 1960s, future issues and directions for public mental health cannot be divorced from the pessimism and mood of retrenchment of the 1980s.

FUTURE DIRECTIONS FOR SERVICE DELIVERY

The major service delivery innovation of the past 25 years has, of course, been CMHCs. Wagenfeld and Jacobs (Chapter 3, this volume) have referred to CMHCs as a "movement"—an organized effort to change some aspect of the social structure perceived to be deficient or defective. Social movements are characterized by leadership, an ideology that spells out the nature of the problem and some goals for remediation, and an organization to carry them out. In speaking of social movements, sociologists and political scientists frequently point to their "natural history"—the phases or stages of their development. Social movements have their origins in an initial unroot or realization that something is wrong with the system. This gradually coalesces into an organized effort at change. At this stage intellectual, often charismatic leaders emerge to define the issues and articulate an ideology. For community mental health, a major figure was Robert Felix, the first director of the NIMH. Another was Gerald Caplan, founder of the Laboratory of Community Psychiatry at Harvard. This early leadership sounds the call to action, defining goals and strategies, and helps generate an enthusiasm and esprit de corps.

As a social movement, community mental health was probably unique in having federal sponsorship and funding almost from the beginning. As the movement grows and matures, as it begins to achieve its early goals, it becomes a part of the established structure. For CMHCs, the availability of large amounts of federal money helped insure rapid expansion. They quickly became part of the service delivery system; they became "institutionalized."[1] Their need for a "voice" helped lead to the establishment of their major professional group, the National Council of Community Mental Health Centers. With inclusion in the social structure of the community, and with the early goals achieved, a movement's leadership and ideology often change, with maintenance, bureaucratization, and survival frequently emerging as major goals. Early aims are reevaluated and modified, even dropped as "unrealistic" or "unfeasible." In this phase of "maturation," the movement becomes part of the established order. As such, it can be a legitimate target for reformers.[2] The attacks on community mental health for being too medical and for not being medical enough, and the changes proposed by the President's Commission on Mental Health (1978) are illustrative of this.

An assessment of the future of mental health services requires that we consider both the accomplishments and failings of CMHCs. There is no gainsaying that the centers have become an established part of the mental health delivery system. They have succeeded in serving large numbers of previously underserved persons and have made substantial progress in redressing the imbalance that previously existed. As such, they are clearly a major part of the mental health delivery system for the foreseeable future.

That they have not succeeded in eliminating war, poverty, sexism, and racism, considered as etiological factors of mental disorders in the period of high enthusiasm when the CMHC was invented, is unfortunate but not surprising. In this sense, the "failure" of community mental health is a reflection of a larger problem in public mental health: an inability to define the nature of its subject matter. This is a point we will consider later. It should be noted that many of the architects of community mental health were also unclear about the meaning of "community." It was assumed that any aggregate of 75,000-200,000 persons would be a community in the sociological sense, that is, having a consciousness of kind, patterns of interaction, institutions, and so on. Leighton (1981) has characterized NIMH's use of community as an "idealized myth."

The report of the President's Commission on Mental Health and, later, the Mental Health Systems Act, reaffirmed the principle of community-based services but called for a more flexible and responsive service system. The notion of a fixed number of services was replaced by community determination of the number and kind of services to be offered. To provide more focus, on the other hand, traditionally underserved groups were targeted for particular attention. This seems to be an improvement, both allowing the community to choose among its possible appropriate services and also emphasizing probable, generally recurring needs.

Another shortcoming of the CMHC program was its failure to generate epidemiological studies of mental disorder. Since centers were established in terms of catchment areas, such investigations would have been relatively simple to launch. This lack of research stemmed from early decisions by the NIMH to subordinate these activities in favor of service delivery. It may not be too cynical to suggest that this could have been done with an eye toward impressing Congress with the volume of services rendered.

With block grants, the direct role of the NIMH in defining programs of CMHCs will be at an end. As Ozarin (Chapter 2, this volume) has noted, it will largely serve an advisory and consultative role in the area of service delivery. States will assume more control or direction over mental health services. The existence of 50 state mental health authorities makes the prediction of future patterns rather chancy. However much the NIMH may have been justifiably critized for failing to give coherent direction and leadership to the CMHC program, it seems difficult to imagine that the current situation is likely to result in increased coherence. One can imagine fierce intrastate competition for scarce resources, with a variety of different types of mental health programs resulting from differently perceived state needs.

From the chapters presented here, several other trends seem within the realm of possibility. CMHCs developed largely as a result of the failures of custodial hospitals. The deinstitutionalization movement, as described by Gruenberg (Chapter 13, this volume), has moved the locus of care into the community. The resulting reduction in the state hospital census, which had begun some eight years before the CMHC legislation as a result of advances in psychopharmacology and changes in the Social Security legislation, was accelerated. In some respects, deinstitutionalization proponents were naive in believing that the chronic patients who had experienced social breakdown as a result of their hospitalization could be moved into the community without extensive support and rehabiliation services. As Gruenberg noted, moving the chronically ill from the long-term hospital to nursing homes or "welfare hotels" was certainly no therapeutic advance. The belated recognition of the needs of these patients was one of the concerns of the PCMH and the Mental Health Systems Act. Stung by what Hollister (Chapter 11, this volume) aptly phrased "the catastrophe of premature deinstitutionalization," concern has been shifting from "pill-centered" aftercare to community support programs for the chronically disabled.

It was noted earlier that in spite of their shortcomings, CMHCs had achieved some notable accomplishments. In a similar fashion, the state hospitals, in spite of serious deficits, perform a useful function. The experiences of the last 25 years indicate that for some percentage of patients, long-term care in a place of refuge or asylum, or the ability to return there for brief periods of restitution, is necessary. Some version of such a facility seems necessary and a likely part of any future delivery system. The rise of vocal patient advocacy groups, alterations of the legal code, a better-trained cadre of mental health personnel, advances in psychopharmacology and rehabilitation techniques, and changes in public consciousness all combine to make very unlikely a return to the isolated custodial hospitals of past decades. But it does seem reasonable to suggest that in a climate of fiscal scarcity, hospitalization may be increasingly viewed as more cost effective and thus desirable. If one adds to this the tendency, in conservative times, to view the cause of social problems as the result of personal rather than societal defects, there may be an added ideological support for hospitalization. The rhetorical excesses of the early leaders of community mental health consigned the long-term hospital to the ash heap of history. But its obituary may have been premature.

Another important issue in service delivery is the realtionship between health and mental health services. In view of the epidemiological evidence that a majority of mental health service are rendered in the general medical sector, the competition for scarce resources, and the ubiquitous pressures for cost effectiveness, continued arguments for a completely separate mental health system seem unlikely to prevail. The PCMH and the Mental Health Systems Act both called for closer ties between the two systems. This philosophy has been continued by the present administration. As Coleman (Chapter 12, this volume) has shown, a variety of models that link mental health and health services exist and are being used. This integration is likely to be much more the norm, or at least the stated goal, in the near future and is likely to be facilitated by an increasing "mainstreaming" of mental health into medicine.

Many of the psychiatric critiques of community mental health (e.g., Borus, 1978; Zusman & Lamb, 1977) have argued that community mental health went too far in the direction of social etiologies and social action. Community mental health was seen as "demedicalized" and "deprofessionalized." What is needed is a "return to basics," that is, the delivery of mental health services to the severely disordered in a medical/psychiatric framework. This is clearly compatible with the increasing pressures for services integration. The pressure to make medical practice more "holistic" will, it is hoped, also enlarge the viewpoint of medicine.

Although one of the original aims of the community mental health program had been to improve services to minorities, continued inadequacies are likely to haunt public mental health for some time to come. Studies over a number of years have documented that minority clients receive discriminatory treatment from white therapists (Lerner, 1971; Padilla et al., 1975; Riessman et al., 1964; D. W. Sue, 1978; Willie et al., 1973). Discrimination could be seen in intake and assignment practices, culturally inappropriate treatment modalities, and poorer treatment outcomes.

Schofield's (1964) famous "YAVIS syndrome" has been cited as one factor behind discriminatory treatment and poorer outcomes. He found that therapists tend to prefer *Y*oung, *a*ttractive, *v*erbal, *i*ntelligent, and *s*uccessful individuals for clients. D. W. Sue (1978) noted that "counselors tend to respond according to their own conditioned values, assumptions and perspectives of reality without regard for other views." He identified four world views represented by clients and therapists based on locus of control and locus of responsibility. He suggested that the internal locus of control and responsibility worldview is most characteristic of Western counseling approaches, but is not typical of many minority clients. Early termination and ineffective outcomes may result.

Levine and Padilla (1980) have pointed out that poor Hispanics are overrepresented for alcohol and drug convictions and underrepresented in mental health facilities. They contended that the poor are often incarcerated for the same behaviors for which the more affluent receive medical and psychiatric help.

In proposing more responsive services for minorities, Stanley Sue (1977) suggested the development of three models of service delivery: modified and upgraded existing services, independent but parallel services, and new nonparallel services. He writes: "A time may well come when minority clients receive equal but unresponsive services and that primary attention should be placed upon the delivery of responsive services rather than upon the demonstration of inequities." Community mental health centers, in other words, should be flexible in regard to services for minorities and develop whatever model is most responsive and provides the best outcome.

A final issue that will most likely have significant impact on service delivery in the coming decades is pattern of funding. The freedom to develop community-based services was, to a considerable extent, afforded by the financial largesse of Congress under the leadership of Senator Hill and Representative Fogarty during the period of most rapid expansion, and to similar generosity of later administrations. As Wagenfeld and Jacobs (Chapter 3, this volume) have noted in their section on legislative history, it was federal funds that made possible the startling changes in pattern of care and the greatly expanded number and sorts of personnel occupied in the care of the mentally disordered. Gruenberg (Chapter 13, this volume), too, noted the changes in the Social Security legislation that helped make possible the release of many patients from mental hospitals.

Additionally, the CMHC legislation changed intergovernmental relationships. Prior to 1963, federal involvement in mental health was almost entirely through direct linkage with the state mental health authorities. After passage of the CMHC legislation, the relationship was between the federal government (NIMH) and local mental health boards. The Omnibus Reconciliation Act of 1981, authorizing block grants, has restored the previous federal/state relationship.

At the end of this almost 30-year period of expansion, it remains to be seen how many of the new sort of services, mostly developed by CMHCs and by general hospital administrators and practitioners, will be able to survive under the pressure of reduced federal funding and leadership. A key here is third-party payment, the extent to which insurance companies and other carriers are willing to reimburse for mental health services. If payment is available only for secondary and tertiary care, where will support come from for preventive and educational efforts? Will state and county governments be able to underwrite the cost of these services? Another uncertainty is the form that will be taken by the administration's concern with escalating hospital costs. What kind of "caps" or changes in reimbursement will be enacted? These are very significant questions, the answers to which will be crucial for the delivery of mental health services in the future.

SOME ISSUES FOR EPIDEMIOLOGY

As Regier's (Chapter 4, this volume) review has shown, the past 25 years in psychiatric epidemiology have seen significant advances in our understanding of mental disorders. The genetic approach has underscored the importance of heritability in the major psychoses. Sociocultural approaches, focusing on global measures of psychological impairment, have explored the significance of such factors as poverty, socioeconomic status, and stress. These approaches by themselves, however, have not succeeded in providing definitive data on etiologies. Psychosocial impairment scales have also failed to relate to clinical diagnostic categories or to provide incidence measures crucial to understanding etiology.

The past quarter-century has also seen advances in clinical psychiatry in the areas of psychopharmacology, neurophysiology, and genetics that have broadened our understanding of mental disorders. DSM-III represents a new, operationalizable approach to diagnosis and classification, and field instruments such as the Diagnostic Interview Schedule (DIS) offer an opportunity for linking epidemiological and clinical levels of observation. With the DIS, data on both the incidence and prevalence of major DSM-III categories of disorder in the community can be obtained. The Epidemiological Catchment Area (ECA) program funded by the NIMH–using the DIS–will provide an ongoing source of data on the incidence and prevalence of mental disorders in both institutionalized and noninstitutionalized populations. There has been insufficient experience with the DIS to draw any conclusions about its efficacy, but it is clear that the "third generation" of instruments in psychiatric epidemiology will have to be standardized and linked to clinical categories in order to permit the application of epidemiological findings to the planning of services. This would certainly aid in the acceptance and utilization of epidemiological findings–a concern expressed by Sartorius.

MANPOWER AND TRAINING DEVELOPMENT

A number of chapters in this volume have touched on changes in manpower needs in the past 25 years. At the beginning of this period, the major mental health resource personnel were psychiatrists, psychologists, psychiatric social workers, and nurses. The shift from institutional care to community care helped to create a need for more persons in these disciplines, as well as for professional staff in various rehabilitation specialties. In the immediate post-World War II period, many training activities were funded by the VA. Later, the NIMH assumed a leadership role.

In the early years of community mental health, public health nurses played a significant role. Unlike other practitioners, they did some of their work in the home, where they were able to observe much of the psychosocial stress that was presumed to be associated with mental disorder. Considerable effort was devoted to producing public mental health nurse consultants, hoping to increase the efficiency of the public health nurse by adding mental to the other health services for families. It is not entirely clear why this effort declined, but it may have been related to a more general shift of attention away from the development of local health departments. At about the same time, the nurse especially trained to care for psychiatric patients and to stand as a full member of the treatment team was emerging.

In addition to public health nursing, two other professional groups initially involved in public mental health have become less prominent. The first is pediatrics. When the child guidance clinic movement was begun about 1920, the pediatrician was an integral member of the psychiatrist/social worker/psychologist team. This did not last long, but it did produce a new subspecialty, exemplified by Spock, Senn, and others. This group was, for a period, most influential—witness the "bible" of child care produced by Spock. Pediatrics also adopted a shared concern with mental health in the area of mental retardation.

Child psychiatry, developed primarily as a source for leadership of child guidance clinic teams, was for a long period the major focus for the development of concepts of prevention in psychiatry in general. With the rapid growth of CMHCs, child psychiatry went into eclipse for a period. Specific concern for the mental health of children by mental health centers was targeted in 1978 as one of the recommendations of the PCMH. Unfortunately, there was not enough time for a strong renascence of the specialty before funding was reduced.

The 1960s saw the emergence of a new occupational category in the health and human services field: the indigenous nonprofessional, or paraprofessional. Although there had been a long tradition of employing nonprofessionals in the mental health field as orderlies or aides, the paraprofessional of the 1960s was different.[3] By coming from the ranks of the poor and minorities, they would, in Pearl and Reissman's (1965) term, "humanize" the delivery of human services and sensitize the largely white, middle-class professionals to the culture and problems of their clients. In an effort to stimulate their development and to credential them, the NIMH supported many training programs, first at the associate level and later at the baccalaureate and master's levels. While some of the romantic aura has subsided, they have become an established part of the mental health care system. With increasing competition for jobs, however, their continued viability may be questioned.

Professional training of health officers to be competent as planners and administrators of mental health services was a goal of the NIMH for a time in the late 1950s and early 1960s. Grants to schools of public health supported faculties in mental health for a period. When funds were withdrawn, most schools were left with small, residual programs in mental health or included mental health as part of the programs in departments of behavioral science. The general attack on social science research by the government may result in further constriction of support for mental health training in schools of public health.

The availability of federal support has, of course, impacted heavily on professional education in the core mental health disciplines. In addition to training large numbers of staff for the CMHCs, federal dollars helped to facilitate the introduction of new curricula in social and community psychiatry and community psychology, as well as in techniques of consultation and education. This federal support also helped to encourage curricular innovations designed to sensitize students to the culture and needs of minorities. This was related to the recognition, noted earlier, that these groups were frequently unserved or underserved.

In addition to educating service deliverers, widespread federal support encouraged research training in psychiatry, the behavioral sciences, epidemiology, and many of the biological sciences. Every indication now is that support for service delivery training and much of research training is at an end. How the training of future cadres of mental health service providers and researchers will be financed is not at all clear at this point.

PREVENTION OF MENTAL DISORDERS

As was pointed out earlier, many of the early leaders of the community mental health movement vastly oversold its potential, claiming that it could do far more than it was actually capable of accomplishing. This was particularly true with respect to the prevention of mental disorders. Using the triumphs of the environmental sanitarians of the 19th century as a model, it was argued that removing the "psychic sewerage" in the environment would accomplish the same reduction in the incidence of mental disorder that was brought about with respect to infectious disease by cleaning up the water supply and environment. The global nature of the claims, vague methodologies, and the misapplication of clinical principles and models resulted in an erosion of the credibility of prevention as a strategy. However, as the Lemkau and Justice chapters have shown, clear specification of the dependent variable, focused interventions, and rigorous methodologies have demonstrated the clear viability of prevention as a goal of public mental health. The two frameworks presented here differ in their focus, but they share a common concern with scientific rigor.

THE NATURE OF MENTAL HEALTH AND MENTAL DISORDER

A persistent, significant, and highly troublesome problem for public mental health and one that is dealt with in different ways in most of these chapters–is the lack of clarity about the definition of the dependent variable: What is meant by "mental health" and "mental illness"? It should be clear from previous chapters that the question is of more than academic interest. Many of the problems encountered by the CMHCs were related to these issues. If community mental health was criticized for attempting to be all things to all people, this could be seen as stemming, in part, from a lack of agreement on the nature of the dependent variable. Calls for the prevention of the amorphous category of "mental disorder" and the promotion of "mental health" and "happiness" created some serious problems for priority setting, resource allocation, and ultimately, credibility.

Gerald Klerman (1979), while administrator of the Alcohol, Drug Abuse, and Mental Health Administration, suggested some of the boundaries of mental health. Essentially, he argued that the treatment of severe mental illness be its central concern. By concentrating on definable disorders–a significant public health problem by any standard–one avoids the difficulties inherent in the vague, amorphous term "mental health." Some of the same concerns expressed by Klerman were also voiced by the Joint Commission on Mental Illness and Health years before in their report, *Action for Mental Health,* in 1961. This volume was one of the strong influences that helped shape the original community mental health legislation. Parenthetically, Leighton (1981) has noted that the myth is not that of mental illness, but of mental health.

Klerman argued further that mental health had several overlapping boundaries that should be recognized by planners and service providers. These boundaries related to distinctions between the enhancement of potential and the seeking of fulfillment versus the treatment of seriously disabling illness and the extent of the societal mandate for mental health interventions.

The epilogue to this volume is not the place to attempt a definitive resolution of the issue of definitions and boundaries. It is appropriate, however, to note its existence as a problem and to suggest that some attention to it be part of public mental health's agenda for the future.

AN AGENDA FOR PUBLIC MENTAL HEALTH

In this chapter we have taken a very broad approach in attempting to describe the accomplishments of public mental health in the past quarter-century and to discerning some future trends. Drawing these together, what agenda can be set for the field for the remainder of the century?

It would seem that the first order of business should be a serious attempt at developing or defining the boundaries of public mental health. This goal, while not unique with us, nonetheless presents a crucial task. It seems difficult to imagine advances in the field when basic issues of definition have not been resolved. Perhaps the vague connotation of the term "mental health" itself is a major part of the problem. From an ideological point of view, "health" is a useful term; for scientific purposes, however, it is less desirable. Perhaps, as both Klerman (1979) and Leighton (1981) have noted, advances in diagnosis and psychopharmacology have made "mental illness" a more defensible focus. This is not antithetical to the historic purposes of public health, nor is a rejection of a population focus, but a clearer definition of the boundaries of the field would enhance both its credibility and its scientific status.

Following this would be the acquisition of a strong data base in epidemiology. As noted, the DIS or other standardized instrument holds some promise in that direction.

With accurate data on incidence and prevalence, a more rational approach to the setting of priorities and planning of services can be developed. As Sartorius (Chapter 6, this volume) has pointed out, the existence of scientifically accurate epidemiological data is not a sufficient condition for its being employed by planners and policy makers. In a pluralistic society, the setting of health and human services policy is never an entirely rational process, in the sense that the data "speak for themselves." It is a political process, and the degree to which interest groups can organize and mobilize frequently influences the ultimate allocation of resources. We have seen how this has been—and most certainly will continue to be—the case with mental health.

However, if mental health services are to be more than simply reactive to transient fads and pressures, priority setting is necessary. The basic issue here is: What should be the major concern of the public mental health system? If, as Kramer (Chapter 5, this volume) has predicted, we are faced with the prospect of a sharp increase in the prevalence of serious mental disorder, then just how these persons are to be served is of utmost concern.

Establishing priorities for service populations will, to a large extent, influence the future of the public mental hospital. It seems clear that deinstitutionalization cannot stand alone as a goal, but rather that it requires extended services in the community. What is necessary is an upgraded network of public mental hospital services linked to the community mental health services system. The role and nature of the state hospital, then, should be an agenda item for public mental health.

The priority-setting process will also help to determine the extent to which mental health becomes "mainstreamed" into the general medical sector. We have pointed out earlier that there seems little likelihood of a continuation of mental health as a totally separate system of care. It would be extreme, however, to envisage a complete merger. The strong tradition of input from the social and behavioral sciences precludes this.

One of the major contributions of the social and behavioral sciences has been the recognition that mental health (or mental disorder), more than other areas in the medical field, is intimately tied up with the value systems of both clients and practitioners. Part of both the purpose and the success of community mental health has been the push toward correcting the imbalance in the service delivery system that largely denied adequate care to minorities and the poor. There has been an increased awareness of the need to provide services in a culturally syntonic manner and to recruit members of racial and ethnic minorities to the mental health disciplines. If the mental health system is to continue over the coming decades in the direction of responsiveness, manpower and training issues must be part of that agenda.

Finally, we have noted that two of the raisons d'être of public health have been the prevention of disorder and the promotion of health. As evidenced by chapters by Lemkau and Justice, respectively, there is considerable disagreement about the appropriate conceptual model for prevention. Whether the most fruitful approach is the prevention of specific, lifecycle-related disorders or the enhancement of coping, social support, and adaptational skills depends to some extent on the nature of the paradigm of disorder that emerges as part of the process of definition and priority setting that we have sketched out. Additionally, public mental health must confront the essentially ideological or political question of the kinds of societal change necessary to prevent stress-induced pathological feelings and behavior. How much change can be made, and what kind of "trade-offs" are involved?

In prevention research, priorities have to be set. Should efforts be directed first to research in brain physiology, research on the mechanisms by which stress acts to change the way the C.N.S. functions, or research to determine the most symptom-provoking kinds of stress? It is clear that agreement exists that efforts at preventing disorder—however defined—must be part of a public mental health agenda and be based on rigorous scientific criteria.

In attempting to divine the future, certain things seem clear. That changes will come in methods of payment for services is obvious. That the mix of kinds of helping people will change is no less apparent. That methods of research will change and develop is also clear. Perhaps the only thing that we can be sure about is that things will not stay the same. Change will come. The hope is that skilled, ethical, and concerned professionals and an alert population will continue to be available for the future development of mental health services for those who need them.

Notes

1. It should be noted that sociologically, "institutionalized" does not have a pejorative connotation. It refers to something being an accepted part of the social structure.

2. The history of public mental health as presented here indicates that this same series of phases applies equally well to an earlier mental health innovation: the state hospital. Established in the early years of the 19th century as an optimistic reform, by the latter part of the century the hospitals had become human warehouses.

3. It is an interesting comment on occupational development and the movement toward professionalism that the paraprofessionals have acquired many of the characteristics of established occupations or disciplines: national organizations, newsletters, and so forth. Their section in the APHA is called "New Professionals."

References

BORUS, J. Issues critical to the survival of community mental health. *American Journal of Psychiatry*, 1978, *135*, 1029-1031.

Joint Commission on Mental Illness and Health. *Action for mental health.* New York: Basic Books, 1961.

KLERMAN, G. The limits of mental health. Paper presented to the Western Psychiatric Institute, Pittsburgh, 1979.

LEIGHTON, A. H. *New England Journal of Human Services,* 1981, *1,* 6-14.

LERNER, B. *Therapy in the ghetto: Political power and personal disintegration.* Baltimore: Johns Hopkins University Press, 1971.

LEVINE, E. S., & PADILLA, A. M. *Crossing cultures in therapy: Pluralistic counseling for the Hispanic.* Monterey, CA: Brooks/Cole, 1980.

PADILLA, A. M., RUIZ, R. A., & ALVAREZ, R. Community mental health services for the Spanish-speaking surnamed population. *American Psychologist,* 1975, *30,* 892-905.

PEARL, A., & REISSMAN, F. *New careers for the poor.* New York: Free Press, 1965.

President's Commission on Mental Health. *Report to the President.* Washington, DC: Government Printing Office, 1978.

RIESSMAN, F., COHEN, J., & PEARL, A. (Eds.) *Mental health of the poor.* New York: Free Press, 1964.

SCHOFIELD, W. *Psychotherapy: The purchase of friendship.* Englewood Cliffs, NJ: Prentice-Hall, 1964.

SUE, D. W. Eliminating cultural oppression in counseling: Toward a general theory. *Journal of Counseling Psychology,* 1978, *25,* 419-428.

SUE, S. Community mental health services to minority groups. *American Psychologist,* 1977, *32,* 616-624.

WILLIE, C., KRAMER, B., & BROWN, B. *Racism and mental health.* Pittsburgh: University of Pittsburgh Press, 1973.

YANAMOTO, J., JAMES, Q. C., & PALLEY, N. Cultural problems in psychiatric therapy. *Archives of General Psychiatry,* 1968, *19,* 45-49.

ZUSMAN, J., & LAMB, H. R. In defense of community mental health. *American Journal of Psychiatry,* 1977, *134*(8), 887-890.

About the Editors

Morton O. Wagenfeld, Ph.D., is Professor of Sociology and Health and Human Services at Western Michigan University, Kalamazoo. He received his Ph.D. in sociology from Syracuse University and underwent postgraduate training in community mental health at the Laboratory of Community Psychiatry, Harvard Medical School. He is a past chairman of the Mental Health Section of the American Public Health Association. His professional interests include epidemiology, mental health delivery systems, and health policy.

Paul V. Lemkau, M.D., is certified by the American Boards of Psychiatry and Neurology and of Preventive Medicine and Public Health. He joined the faculty of the Johns Hopkins University School of Hygiene and Public Health in 1939 and became the first Professor and Chairman of its Department of Mental Hygiene in 1961. He has done extensive studies of the epidemiology of mental disorders in the United States and Yugoslavia and has served as a World Health Organization consultant in Yugoslavia, Japan, Venezuela, Surinam, and India.

Blair Justice, Ph.D., is a Professor of Psychology at the University of Texas School of Public Health in Houston. He is the author of three books and many articles on family violence, stress and coping, and related subjects. He is a past chairman of the Mental Health Section of the American Public Health Association and is on the editorial board of the *International Journal of Mental Health.* He is also a member of the Psychiatric Residency Program faculty at the Texas Research Institute of

Mental Sciences and a Faculty Associate at the University of Texas Center for Health Promotion, Research and Development.

About the Contributors

Jules V. Coleman, M.D., is currently Clinical Professor Emeritus of Psychiatry and Public Health, as well as Lecturer in Psychiatry, at Yale University. From 1962 to 1972 he headed the Mental Health Section of the Department of Epidemiology and Public Health at the Yale School of Medicine. He also served as Chief, Mental Health and Psychiatry, of the Community Health Care Center in New Haven, Connecticut, from 1972 to 1979 and in 1974 received the Annual Award of the Mental Health Section of the American Public Health Association.

Ernest M. Gruenberg, M.D., Dr.P.H., was Professor and Chairman of the Department of Mental Hygiene, Johns Hopkins School of Hygiene and Public Health from 1975 to 1981. His first achievement in the field of public health was the formulation of the New York State Mental Health Act (1954), which opened the field of local government community psychiatry. He chaired the APHA Program Area Committee on Mental Health, which produced the 1962 Mental Disorder Control Methods and introduced the concept that the Chronic Social Breakdown Syndrome is largely preventable. Currently, he is Co-Principal Investigator for the Eastern Baltimore Mental Health Survey, a major mental health survey underway at Johns Hopkins.

William G. Hollister, M.D., is currently Professor Emeritus of Community Psychiatry at the University of North Carolina, School of Medicine. His interests and writings have been in the training of consultation to executive staff of mental health centers in methods of alternative care in school and rural mental health, prevention, interagency consultation, and mental health education. He is a former chief of Community Research & Services of the National Institute of Mental Health.

Judith H. Jacobs, Dr. P.H., is currently a Research Scientist, Division of Biometry and Epidemiology, at the National Institute of Mental Health. Before that she was Acting Chief of the Mental Health Services Support Branch that oversaw the CMIIC program. She has taught at The Johns Hopkins University, Temple University, Harvard University, and the University of Massachusetts.

Morton Kramer, Sc.D., is Professor of Mental Hygiene at The Johns Hopkins University, School of Hygiene and Public Health. Prior to this appointment he was Chief of the National Institute of Mental Health's Biometrics Branch, from 1949 to 1975, and Director of the Division of Biometry and Epidemiology, from 1975 to 1976. He has written extensively on the application of biostatistical and epidemiological methods to research on the prevention and control of mental disorders in the United States and other countries of the world.

Alan David Miller, M.D., is currently Associate Dean of Student Affairs, Clinical Professor of Psychiatry, and Professor of Community and Preventive Medicine at the Albany Medical College. He is certified by the American Board of Psychiatry and Neurology. From 1966 to 1975 he was Commissioner of the New York State Department of Mental Hygiene. He was a member of the National Advisory Mental Health Council from 1969 to 1973 and participated in the first U.S. Mental Health Mission to the Soviet Union in 1967. He is on the editorial boards of *Psychiatric Quarterly* and *Administration in Mental Health.*

Lucy D. Ozarin, M.D., is currently a Psychiatric Consultant at the National Institute of Mental Health. From 1957 to 1981 she served as Program Development Officer at the NIMH. She is a Fellow of the American Public Health Association and of the

American College of Physicians. She received her psychiatric training at Grasslands Hospital, Westchester County, New York, and at the Washington-Baltimore Psychoanalystic Institute.

Nolan E. Penn, Ph.D., is a Professor of Psychiatry at the University of California at San Diego, School of Medicine, La Jolla. He is Director of Community and Forensic Psychiatry Training programs in the Psychiatry Department. In addition, he is the Medical Schools Regional Director for the Area Health Education Centers System, a program that seeks to direct 10 percent of medical-clinical training hours into underserved areas in both urban and rural geographic regions. His responsibilities in the general health care delivery field also keep him in touch with training and workforce distribution issues regarding mental health care delivery.

Darrel A. Regier, M.D., has been Director of the Division of Biometry and Epidemiology, National Institute of Mental Health, since 1977. The division supports both intramural and extramural research programs in epidemiology, mental health services systems research, statistics, and clinical services research. He has published approximately 20 scientific articles and is currently a member of the American Psychiatric Association, the American Public Health Association, the International Epidemiologic Association, and the World Psychiatric Association Section Steering Committee on Community and Epidemiologic Psychiatry.

Dwight W. Rieman, M.S.W., is currently an Associate Professor in the School of Social Work at the University of Missouri-Columbia. He directed two three-year, NIMH-supported, continued education projects for Missouri mental health facilities, one on consultation, the other on staff board collaboration in community mental health programs. He has had extensive urban and rural experience in mental health, including the areas of direct service, supervision, consultation, community organization, administration, and education.

Norman Sartorius, M.D., Ph.D., is Director of the Division of Mental Health, World Health Organization, and Professor of Transcultural Psychiatry at the University of Zagreb, Yugoslavia. He holds degrees in medicine and psychology and has published more than 100 articles and books. His research interests include the cross-cultural and epidemiological aspects of mental health, the evaluation of mental health care, and methodology in the behavioral sciences.